6-18-69

Health Is a Community Affair

Health Is a
Community Affair

REPORT OF THE NATIONAL COMMISSION

ON COMMUNITY HEALTH SERVICES

HARVARD UNIVERSITY PRESS

Cambridge, Massachusetts 1967

Distributed in Great Britain by Oxford University Press, London
Library of Congress Catalog Card Number 66-27415
Printed in the United States of America

The publication of this volume has been aided
by a grant from The Commonwealth Fund

To the People of the United States:

It is my privilege and great honor to present to you this report, called *Health Is a Community Affair*. It is my wish and that of my colleagues that this particular affair may prosper in communities all over the land — that the findings and recommendations so carefully considered here will give inspiration and guidance to community leadership everywhere.

The National Commission on Community Health Services is a private corporation, sponsored by the American Public Health Association and the National Health Council. It has conducted in the past four years a nationwide study of community health needs, resources, and practices. It remains now for you to translate the Commission's studies into action.

This report is a synthesis of six task force explorations and a report on community action studies drawn from 21 communities extending across the country from Springfield, Massachusetts, to San Mateo, California, and ranging in population from 30,000 to 3,500,-000. The report also considers papers from the White House Conference of 1965, other health studies (community and national), and the health legislation that has been enacted into law during the life of the Commission.

The Commission has earnestly sought to incorporate into its recommendations the thought and experience of citizens with wide-ranging responsibilities and interests. They are deeply concerned with health and with the urgency of closing the gap between what we know in the health sciences and what we do about preventing health hazards which threaten the life of modern man. These citizens are lawyers, physicians, educators, engineers, salesmen, housewives, and politicians. They represent a fair cross section of this country's community leadership.

The work of the Commission has been made possible by contributions from private foundations, industry, government, and business.

We address this report to you in the full knowledge that quality health services for all the people will require responsible action by individuals, by communities, and by health agencies serving in every dimension of public and private life.

April 22, 1966

Sincerely yours,
Marion B. Folsom
CHAIRMAN

National Commission on Community Health Services

SPONSORS

The American Public Health Association
National Health Council

OFFICERS

Marion B. Folsom, M.B.A., LL.D., Chairman
James E. Perkins, M.D., Dr.P.H., Vice-Chairman
Joseph L. Beesley, C.L.U., Treasurer
Dean W. Roberts, M.D., M.P.H., Secretary

COMMISSIONERS

C. H. Hardin Branch, M.D.
LeRoy Collins, LL.B.
Nelson H. Cruikshank, B.D.
Fairleigh S. Dickinson, Jr.
Stanford F. Farnsworth, M.D., M.P.H.
Harry G. Hanson, M.S.
Harold A. James, Ph.B., LL.B.
John W. Knutson, D.D.S., Dr.P.H.
William F. McGlone, LL.B.
Joseph H. McNinch, M.D.
Peter G. Meek (ex officio)
Charles D. Shields, M.D., M.P.H.
Virginia Dodd Smith, A.B.
John H. Venable, M.D., M.P.H.
Raymond L. White, M.D.

Leroy E. Burney, M.D., M.P.H.
Edwin L. Crosby, M.D., Dr.P.H.
Albert W. Dent, LL.D.
Milton Stover Eisenhower, LL.D., D.Sc.
James A. Hamilton, M.C.S.
Herman E. Hilleboe, M.D., M.P.H.
Boisfeuillet Jones, B.Ph., LL.B.
Sanford P. Lehman, M.D., M.P.H.
Walter J. McNerney, M.H.A.
Berwyn F. Mattison, M.D., M.P.H. (ex officio)
Marion W. Sheahan, R.N.
Charles E. Smith, M.D., D.P.H.
William C. Treuhaft, L.H.D.
Jane E. Wrieden, M.S.W.

COMMITTEE ON THE COMMISSION REPORT

Harold A. James, Ph.B., LL.B., Chairman
Herman E. Hilleboe, M.D., M.P.H.
James E. Perkins, M.D., Dr.P.H.
Marion W. Sheahan, R.N.
Charles D. Shields, M.D., M.P.H.
Raymond L. White, M.D.

Preface

The formation of the National Commission on Community Health Services in September 1962 was a practical response to the demands of health professionals and other civic-minded individuals toward achieving a concerted effort that could cope effectively with new and changing hazards to health, reduce the waste of health service resources, and prepare for the health service demands of the future. The Commission was created by the American Public Health Association and the National Health Council. The sponsors gave the Commission complete freedom to conduct the necessary studies, develop its recommendations, and report to the American people.

The Commission organized its investigation under three projects. Through its National Task Forces Project, it set up six task forces (on Environmental Health; Comprehensive Personal Health Services; Health Manpower; Health Care Facilities; Financing Community Health Services and Facilities; and Organization of Community Health Services), each composed of 10 to 15 members, representing a range of professional skills, backgrounds, and points of view required to insure balanced consideration of six particular subject areas. The members of the task forces were distinguished leaders in their respective fields. They were selected as imaginative thinkers representing a variety of outlooks. The Commission gave the task forces full freedom to pursue their studies and to develop their recommendations with assurance that their reports would be published as finally submitted.

The Commission's second project was built around 21 community self-studies, taking inventories of health services as they now exist, identifying needs for service, suggesting means to establish comprehensive health services, and determining methods of converting plans into action. The Community Action-Studies Project, under the guidance of nationally known experts, studied community health problems through the eyes, ears, and hands of the community leaders. To balance any potential theoretical approach by task forces, the community studies asked what people in local communities saw as their important health problems, how far they themselves could go in evaluating and solving them, and by what methods. At the same time, special studies were undertaken on the process of community action, the "community readiness" factor in successful or unsuccessful community ventures, and the results of previous community health studies. These studies are grouped together under the Commission's Community Action-Studies Project reports. They will be published as they are completed.

The third project was communications. It concerned itself primarily with the National Health Conference in 1965, a *Newsletter* during the four years of the Commission's life, and other publications. The preliminary findings and recommendations of the Community Action Studies and of the six task forces were presented in September 1965 to the National Conference, assembled in four forums, at San Francisco, Chicago, Atlanta, and Philadelphia. Hundreds of health professionals and other community leaders attended these meetings, studied the provisional task force recommendations and community action study findings, and suggested modifications out of their local experience. These were the people who would be called upon to carry out the recommendations in their own communities. Thus, the Commission had before it the reactions and new ideas of a cross section of the nation's health leadership.

This final report of the National Commission on Community Health Services is based, therefore, on the findings and recommendations of these projects, and draws upon professional opinion rather than upon analysis of new data. The Commission reserved the prerogative of developing its own report, but it has borrowed substantially from reports of the task forces and the community studies in preparing that report.

The Commission report is a report for use. It is designed for use by the people in communities of all sizes who work, both professionally and as volunteers, for more effective health services —

housewives, physicians, lawyers, engineers, businessmen, educators, bankers, ministers — representing all the various professions, interests, and responsibilities involved in community health enterprise.

Basically, the report is a set of recommendations developed by the kind of people who will use them. The recommendations support 14 major positions. Each position represents a critical area of concern upon which future health practices must be planned. Some represent advanced concepts in health services; others, well-known concepts which the Commission feels should be more widely accepted.

The final chapter of this book comprises the Commission's positions and recommendations. In that chapter, reference is made to the pages on which these positions and recommendations (frequently paraphrased) appear. Throughout the book, the position or recommendation number is shown in brackets. In effect, the "recommendations" are components of the "positions." For instance, position B points to the necessity of assuring the "availability of personal health services of high quality to all people in each community." The Commission recommendations under position B point to specific actions which would contribute to this availability.

The report does not attempt to be inclusive. It presents neither pattern nor prototype. It was the firm policy of the Commission that its report would raise the critical issues, discuss them, and take unequivocal positions, but would not specify in detail the methods of implementation. This will be the responsibility of the communities.

Communities will develop their individual systems of services, using the recommendations of the report as principles and guides or as statements of policy. The Commission urges only that they be put to use.

Dean W. Roberts, M.D.
EXECUTIVE DIRECTOR AND SECRETARY

Acknowledgments

The Commission is indebted to many people for the production of *Health Is a Community Affair*. It owes its very existence to those farsighted few who conceived the idea of such a private, independent study and made bold advances to secure money with which to support it. Major contributors to the Commission's work were the McGregor Fund, the Kellogg Foundation, the Public Health Service of the United States Department of Health, Education, and Welfare, the Vocational Rehabilitation Administration, the New York Foundation, and the Commonwealth Fund.

Thirty-two busy commissioners gave of their time to this endeavor. Included among them were representatives of the Commission's sponsors: Dr. Berwyn Mattison from the American Public Health Association and Mr. Peter Meek from the National Health Council. Members of three advisory committees, whose chairmen were Dr. Ernest L. Stebbins, Dr. George James, and Mr. Aloys H. Thiemann, six task forces, four regional forum committees, and four community research teams worked on the investigations necessary for this report. Leaders and committee members in 21 communities across the nation put in endless hours on self-studies and the research associated with them. Agencies, both private and governmental, were generous with advice, time, and staff. Particular appreciation should be given to the American Medical Association, the American Hospital Association, and the Public Health Service of the United States Department of Health, Education, and Welfare.

Finally, the Commission staff, which carried the burden of coordinating and focusing all these efforts toward production of this report, deserves special appreciation. The full professional staff is listed elsewhere in this report, but I would here record our particular indebtedness to Dr. Dean W. Roberts, Executive Director of the Commission; T. Lefoy Richman, Assistant Executive Director for Communications; Aaron L. Andrews, Assistant Executive Director for Administration; Walter M. Beattie, Director of the National Task Forces Project; Paul Mico, initial Director of the Community Action-Studies Project, and Lee Holder, his associate, who succeeded him; Dr. Perry F. Prather, Special Consultant to the Executive Director; Richard H. Schlesinger, Associate Director of the Task Forces Project; Wanda Van Goor, Director of Publications; Hazel Holly, writer; Clyde Hall, editor; and an able staff of secretaries and clerical helpers who prepared manuscript many times over.

We acknowledge our gratitude for the investment of time and money this report represents, and we are confident that the investment is a wise one.

Marion B. Folsom
CHAIRMAN

Contents

Health Is a Community Affair

CHAPTER I

Health and the Community

Health services, operated to meet the health needs of every individual, should be located within the environment of the individual's home community. This concept is generally agreed upon today. Agreement on what constitutes "a community" is not so generally accepted.

The concept of a health-services "community" in the last half of the twentieth century is complicated, as witness attempts to describe it with such terms as "health communities," "health trade areas," "health service catchment areas," and "health problem-sheds." No matter what terminology is used to express the concept, the community in modern America has dimensions which cannot be defined merely in terms of plane geometry. We were primarily a rural folk when the United States was young; most of our forebears thought of a piece of land — flat or hilly, wide or high — as home. Later, a street address became the symbol for the places where most of us live, work, and die.

More recent is the realization that a community for any one individual shifts and changes dynamically, as his own movements and his many needs for services are interrelated in his daily living situations. Most American citizens have at least one thing in common: mobility. This here-today-and-gone-tomorrow population is pushing the boundaries established by surveyors and politicians into new forms, so that the shape of a community that exists for one purpose today may not be identical with that of a community organized to meet other needs in other times — say those of the burgeoning railroads in the nineteenth century — even though parts of them, both geographically and politically, may be the same.

The individual, going his daily round, sets the boundaries of his community. If, to secure a product or a service, he crosses a county line, a state line, and returns through still another state, then for him the real community is an intercounty and interstate area. Boundaries, originally established by mountains or rivers and further influenced by canals, turnpikes, and railroads, are now relevant mostly for political purposes. The demands and aspirations of more people within a more affluent society have changed these former concepts of community.

People dealing with community health problems today must orient themselves to living situations in which service patterns change, resources change, and community aspirations change. Coagulations of shops and houses strung solidly along a major transportation artery are in no sense political communities, but in fact they swallow the small towns and change their function. Highway construction is a prime force in this, as is state policy regarding intersections, the location of shops (back from or by the side of the throughway), and other matters involving local, state, and federal interests. The results of these and other factors are that some political communities are lovely places in which to live, and others are behavioral sinks where the stresses of chronic poverty produce breeding grounds for emotional and physical disturbance and disease.

The rate and kinds of change necessary even to approximate the health needs of this country will involve us all for our lifetime. Out of chaos has come a time of crisis, but crisis can be defined as a period or situation which, because of its immediacy, demands and forces decision. In the ideographs of the Chinese language, two characters are used to write the single word "crisis" — one is the character for "danger" and the other is the character for "opportunity."

The Community of Solution

The Commission suggests, on the basis of its studies, that where health services are concerned the boundaries of each community are established by the boundaries within which a problem can be defined, dealt with, and solved. Such communities relating to community health services in the United States today are complex in administrative procedures and in traditionally protective

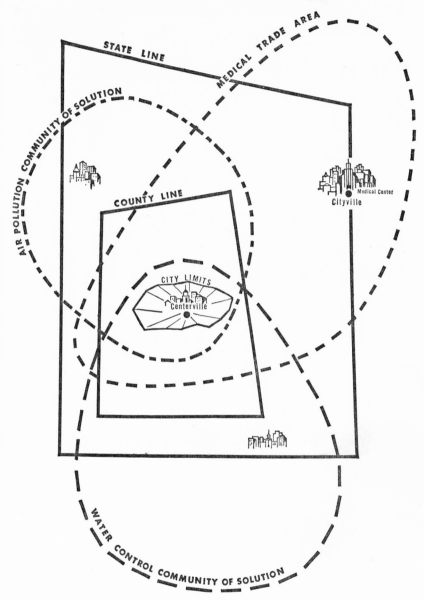

Figure 1. One city's communities of solution. Political boundaries, shown in solid lines, often bear small relation to a community's problem-sheds or its medical trade area.

attitudes toward maintenance of the status quo. Fully aware of the difficulties of arriving at a common point of departure from which improvement of health services can proceed with dispatch and without a total disruption of things as they are, the Commission is convinced that

the planning, organization, and delivery of community health services by both official and voluntary agencies must be based on the concept of a "community of solution" — that is, environmental health problem-sheds and health service marketing areas — rather than primarily on political jurisdictions. [A]

Every political community is a segment of a landmass. Alone it cannot control its water upstream or its air upwind, supply all its needs for health personnel, or finance the wide range of health services scientific advance has made possible. Decisions by other communities, by state or regional or national bodies, affect its actions. Alone it cannot protect its people from health hazards that come from other communities nor, indeed, other countries. Conversely, what it does with its sewage, its votes, its money, or its sick people affects other communities and the nation as a whole.

The predicament suggests its own solution. If single political communities cannot resolve their health problems, they may be able to work them out through revision of existing health jurisdiction boundaries and joint action by several jurisdictions. Compacts and agreements among the various political communities will help speed solution of environmental problems such as the pollution of air and water. Other compacts, agreements, or even complete revisions of jurisdictional boundaries are necessary to administer other high quality health services equally essential to the population.

Administrative and organizational implications of this position (discussed in Chapter VII) are secondary, however, to the understanding and acceptance of the basic concept. It can be repetitively illustrated for public and private agencies. Development of the newer governmental health programs will require substantial increases in health department funds. But budgets are drawn up and adopted by existing political jurisdictions. In practical terms, this financial fact of life may mean reconsideration of budgets and of administrative units providing the health services. For example, a single county health unit, no matter how effective its leadership and how wise its intentions, may lack the population and the financial resources to initiate those health service programs that require many specialties and expensive equipment. As a rule of thumb, a restricted base from which resources can be obtained tends to confine the health department to the provision of the minimum health services.

In the community self-studies which are a part of the Commission's concern, six communities expanded the geographic area of coverage once their studies were under way. These were Knoxville and Chattanooga in Tennessee; Toledo, Ohio; Newark, New Jersey; Springfield, Massachusetts; and Reno, Nevada. Study areas were expanded when, in each of the six communities, the individuals conducting the study found that they were not studying the health needs of the persons involved in the actual health and medical service area. In Reno, Nevada, for example, the study focused on the hospital needs of the people of Reno and its immediately surrounding communities. Analysis of the area showed that, in fact, many of the people receiving hospitalization in Reno came from distant areas in northeastern California and southeastern Oregon. The study personnel then lifted its sights to include the actual service area. A similar situation exists, in terms of hospital use, in Knoxville, Tennessee. Chattanooga found that its community of solution included parts of three states.

There are even some health problems for which the community of solution must be global, such as eradication of smallpox and malaria, uniform definitions and terminology concerning causes of deaths, and international definition and standards for drugs and other therapeutic agents. These must be dealt with through the support of health programs of international agencies (such as the World Health Organization, the United Nations Children's Fund, the World Medical Association, and other nongovernmental international organizations). Through participation in and assistance to international efforts to control disease and raise standards of living, the federal government and the voluntary agencies and societies (such as the national voluntary health agencies through their international counterparts, the American Medical Association through the World Medical Association, and the National Citizens Committee for the World Health Organization) help to protect the health of citizens in all communities. [A-6]

As the center of responsibility for assuring that personal and environmental health services are available to all residents, the community should first assay its resources, its paramount needs, and the strengths that exist to meet those needs. After the community has assessed its resources, it can join with other communities to solve larger problems that require resources of a larger geographical region, a wider political jurisdiction, and more funding than is available to one locality.

Reports of the Commission's community self-studies indicate how new is the concept of interrelated communities and how far we must go before regional planning and action are generally accepted and organized on a routine operational basis. The reports of the Commission task forces also indicate that the idea of separatism has not as yet yielded to the realities of interdependence. In the past, planners in the health field have preferred to operate and to plan independently — hospitals for hospitals, voluntary associations for voluntary associations, health departments for health departments — and even those bold enough to question the wisdom of the system saw little real hope for change.

For health agencies, generally, joint planning has been retarded by fears that such planning mechanisms might bring about "outside control" or loss of identity or autonomy. But the Commission's studies illustrate that a wide range of health agencies can collaborate successfully with other community leadership in planning and action leading toward comprehensive health services — both personal and environmental.

The Web of the Community

Neither communities nor their problems are self-contained. What good are the best of health services if necessary transportation is not available to the person who needs them? Or if these services are beyond the family's financial means? Or if the man who needs them doesn't know they exist? Or if he cannot meet the rules of eligibility to receive them? The fate of the population's health is closely intertwined with issues that have not been identified primarily as health issues. Realistically, health cannot be considered apart from environmental, social, and economic influences. Personal and environmental health services are inextricably intertwined. One lives in an environment of things and people. Whatever a man's genetic inheritance, much of his health is dependent upon the quality of his relation with his environment. The opportunity to work and job security are as essential to man as access to a hospital. Poverty in all its insidious complexities acts like a virus, affecting the health of the total community. Communication and transportation are as necessary for health as the services they summon and deliver.

Each of the Commission's community health studies demonstrates that the level of health services and the level of general community organization are interdependent, driving home the public health aphorism that "the community is the patient." The essential basis for any community's action to supply adequate health services is its economic, political, civic, and professional leadership.

The economic life of the community is usually the focus of primary concern among local leaders. In the United States in the last third of the twentieth century, this concern revolves around the linked processes of urbanization and industrialization. We have become an urban society supported by a complex industrial system; our clustering together in cities and our dependence on that industrial system, complicated by the automation revolution, demand that we be socially inventive and receptive to rapid change. Influential citizens looking at their communities are likely to single out the problems of urbanization as primary: urban renewal; the renovation of the downtown area, which has been subject to decay in most older cities; traffic and parking control; housing.

A revamped urban pattern is currently accepted as a necessity not only for providing an effective, convenient life for the present population, but as a setting for population growth. In particular, there is an urgent sense that the city must offer a scrubbed and attractive face to newcomers, especially to the hoped-for industrial employers who must be lured to the area if its economic vitality is to be sustained. Success in attracting new industry is important to economic life and to the buoyancy of community spirit. The entry of a large, new industrial plant promises employment to many residents; it also gives everyone the feeling that the community is on the move and that other activities, health services included, can go forward.

Political organization also raises problems that are not specifically related to health affairs but are crucial as the setting for health action. Typically, there are four units of increasing size whose mandates for activities of all kinds tend to be unclear, often archaic, and ill-coordinated: those of city or town, county, state, and federal governments. The planning, financing, and operating of health services occur at each of these levels, both in government and in numerous private health agencies.

Especially in small and medium-sized cities, lack of clarity in levels of political organization and responsibility is aggravated by the fear that too many functions now tend to fall into the sphere of the federal government. Feelings of local pride and autonomy are very strong, coupled with the recognition that detailed planning must take into account the unique features of a specific community. Since a large portion of funds available for health care is of federal or state origin, many communities are vexed by the conflict between localism (both as an ideology and to some extent as operational fact) and the necessity for securing significant amounts of federal or state monies.

The relation of broader economic and political problems to health issues is shaped also by results that appear to be more tangible. A person can see a new industry or a revitalized downtown area; he can often assess the impact of a changed political structure. It can be much more difficult to show that the community success in improving the organization of health services is as dramatic and as important.

Underlying the mood of a community's action is its attitude concerning the rights of individuals and groups and their acceptance of each other. This civility of relationships, or its lack, is a significant factor in the health problems of the community. Although racial relations are perhaps the most conspicuous of these problematic features in local life, they are by no means the only ones. Just as interracial hostility or indifference may affect economics, politics, and health care, so a pattern of friction among ethnic groups, socio-economic levels, or subregions of the city may adversely affect concerted community action. In the field of health, where it is so difficult to mobilize diverse local resources, energies required for identifying needs and planning and executing services may be dissipated by the demands of old community antagonisms or claims of competing groups. The coincidence of Negro population density with depressed socio-economic circumstances often means that Negroes form a disproportionate fraction of the medically indigent. If this indigency, with its implicit heavy demands for health care, is compounded by the disadvantage of discriminatory interracial patterns, problems of providing broad scale health care are multiplied.

Health Problems in the Web

Among the problems caught in the web of economics and politics, those primarily identified with the health needs of a community are more starkly visible to the eyes of the health professionals than to the community as a whole. In the community at large, however, these issues vary, both in importance and visibility. Community leaders concerned with health problems have several jobs at hand before they can commence work on the problems themselves. They must first convince the community of the facts of a prevailing health situation, trace the underlying implications of that situation, and in so doing involve the interest of the power leadership within the community in changing the situation.

For instance, although an outbreak of contagious disease may be no respecter of persons and signals loudly for prompt action, the signal will not come through to all residents of the town or city. An epidemic or a continuing health problem such as an outbreak of syphilis or a polluted lake brings many things in its train. Such situations affect public expenditures, which are almost immediately reflected in rising tax rates and other gauges of the community economy; they must also be evaluated in the light of economic stability for the entire population.

The provision of medical care for persons who cannot pay for it may seem at first to be the concern solely of those indigent individuals. To open the eyes of the community leadership and the public, care of the medically indigent must be interpreted in terms of gains and losses — to themselves and to the total community — in a framework of both humanity and economics. Inadequate services to indigent, chronically ill patients or failure to provide rehabilitation services to the disabled may drain productive talent from local industry, as well as freeze potential taxpayers at a low-income rate. Thus, many persons will be unable to earn enough to pay for either their illness or their taxes. Leaders in every town know this; few want to face it.

It is much easier, in presenting health problems to the public, to obtain funds for repairing a faulty sewerage system that can be seen and smelled than it is to sell the same public on the need for concensus in allocating facilities and patients among several local hospitals. The 21 communities in the Commission's Community Action Studies Project worked at these problems over a period of three years. Through self-studies of health services, in cooperation with the Commission, they organized to identify and assess their community health problems, and to set goals, develop plans of action, and (most important) to take corrective or preventive action. Nearly all the study communities exhibit capacity, or potential capacity, to provide better medical care for the total population than that now prevailing. Yet there is a general pattern of overlapping functions, ineffectual use of capacities, and a haphazard provision of service to the people who need it most. The most prominent issue appears to be the need to coordinate facilities to provide care for a variety of illnesses.

Community after community is becoming aware of the need to tie the network of local services together more logically and to plan together to meet health needs already obvious today and likely to confront us for the next several decades. Hearteningly in this morass the community studies are uncovering not only health needs but also health resources that might not otherwise have been discovered. The very assembly of private and public agencies to survey the health of the community opens possibilities for collaboration and creates an interest in achieving more efficient provision of services.

One of the most frequent examples of this in the community studies was the finding that hospital facilities — and professional health manpower — could be reorganized and redistributed to achieve better care for individuals. There is growing recognition that in our highly interdependent modern society, especially within the urban complex, health resources cannot be allowed to grow haphazardly, solely to meet emergency requirements. Some degree of planning, some articulation of people and institutions, certainly seems mandatory. One large community had seven separate hospitals, run by seven separate boards, competing for services, equipment, and recognition. A smaller community, with only two hospitals, had ethnic differences that precluded a close cooperative or coordinative relationship. Another community had four hospitals, each with an electroencephalograph, but only one person in the town was qualified to operate the equipment and interpret its findings. The towns and cities may be different; differences may vary according to race, color, creed, and economic or social status; health problems and resources may differ; but the result is the same throughout the country: costly fragmentation and duplication.

The Commission's 21 communities decided to act, refusing to accept these problems as inevitable. The results of these action studies, carried out locally with resources available to the communities, are impressive — as in the community where the hospital groups are now talking to one another and are starting to plan together, or the community where the hospital boards are cooperating on a joint fund drive for the first time in history. Another community plans a fund drive to improve a medical complex serving the area, adding medical research, medical training, outpatient, and other related services.

In this action-planning process, not all was expansion. One group, after thoughtful study and analysis of all the facts, decided against expansion, canceling plans for a new pediatric hospital in favor of augmenting pediatric services in the existing facilities. Efforts and successes at coordination were not related exclusively to hospital facilities. Some community groups established new regional planning bodies within a multijurisdictional area, regional planning councils, and health councils, as well as health and hospital planning groups. Some groups developed master plans, others, guidelines for agencies to follow as needed.

For years health services have grown as a reaction to crises. Good administrators realize that some crises are inevitable and have capitalized on them to obtain needed services, personnel, or funds. But today more communities and more leaders within them have begun to realize that crisis reaction is inadequate and wasteful. It is more economical, wise, and humane to act to prevent crisis, using voluntary cooperation within the community to anticipate future needs and to prepare to meet them, rather than, by default, to await the imposition of a central design from without.

The Bridge between Knowledge and Practice

There are without doubt in this country sophisticated, learned, and dedicated health professionals, representing all health disciplines and operating in public health departments, voluntary health agencies, professional societies, private practice, academic and research settings, and clinical facilities. In looking toward the horizon of preventive medicine and ideal environments, and in striving for greater perfection in the better-developed areas of the country, these men and women must remember, however, that many communities in the United States as yet do not even possess a local practicing physician, reasonable proximity to a hospital, plumbing beyond the privy, or garbage disposal without rats.

Nevertheless, most community residents expect almost without question certain services: protection from pollution of the environment, a wide range of preventive services, and practical arrangements through which they can obtain high quality health care when ill or injured. Residents moving from home communities where they accepted such services as casually as the mail delivery find them unobtainable in their new homes. Many communities have grown up so fast around metropolitan areas that they lack even the rudimentary tools to obtain these services. Unincorporated areas often are not covered by local regulations, and state regulations, if they exist, go unenforced. Permeating every community's efforts to solve these problems is the frustration which develops out of the inability to cope with many of them without becoming involved in identical problems of the larger region of which the community is a part.

For every community, the problem of health is the problem of people, whether they be too many or too few. Some communities have been almost overwhelmed by newcomers whose current demands on health and other services cannot be met. In Los Angeles these newcomers add at least 3000 automobiles to the city's freeways every month. For other communities, health problems stem from a scarcity of people. Within some counties of Appalachia, lack of job opportunities has caused more than half the residents to migrate to the industrial centers of Ohio and other states. Most of the people who remain in those Appalachian counties are the elderly, who cannot take care of themselves, and the unemployed who receive some form of public assistance. Gone from those hills and hollows are the young married couples and the others who, traditionally, would be providing and financing the necessary services in their community.

Particular communities, then, encounter specific problems indigenous to themselves, but the health problems for every community in the United States have their foundations in current attitudes, knowledge, and aspirations. We have the knowledge to prevent more disease than we prevent today; we have the knowledge to treat more illness than we treat; we know more about controlling environmental health hazards than we put into practice. Recent health legislation is indicative of public impatience with the current situation as well as of the desire of many community leaders and health professionals to improve it. It may be that the fate of the community concept rests, in the last third of the twentieth century, with the initiative displayed by responsible community leaders as they reassess their role in narrowing the gaps between health service potential and current practice.

In attempting to narrow those gaps, communities must not bind themselves by adherence to traditional methods. Just as the community of solution requires an objective appraisal of geographic and political boundaries, so does the delivery of health services require flexibility and experimentation in method. No system of organization or administration should be considered permanent; new ones must be devised — tried, discarded, or developed — to keep pace with changing needs. Communities will reach their goal of comprehensive health services by many different paths and no alternative route should be blocked.

The performance of community health services should not be considered the province solely of the physician and the public health officer. It must be recognized that the health "team" is not a closed fraternity but includes all those who work together to improve the health of people. Individually and collectively, they share this responsibility. The vested interests of voluntary, private, and public agencies and of the professions must be subjugated to the overriding interest — that of the health of people.

It has become fashionable to dismiss much of the community involvement in the manpower problem by stating that the problem is too big for any community to solve and is a national concern, rather than a local one. This is largely but not entirely true, as aggressive communities that have actively recruited health manpower and retained skilled health personnel can testify. In order to attract the bright young men of the newer scientific and industrial professions, many communities emphasize the particular virtues of their region — climate, topography, educational opportunities, or pleasant family settings. Health professionals, like others, are interested in such fringe benefits. Many health workers choose their vocations and professions because they like to help people; they are dedicated to their work and are often more attracted by freedom to pursue it in the way they think best than by higher pay scales. The alert community wishing to employ sufficient health personnel of high quality for its programs can do much toward achieving that objective, but it requires energy, innovation, and determination.

The suggestions offered by communities in the Commission's community studies were similar to those developed by its Task Force on Health Manpower. Among them were: look to unexpected places within your community for leadership, and make greater use of retired persons and nonhealth-oriented persons in planning and other health program activities; make full use of available scholarship and loan programs, and begin recruiting efforts at the early high school level.

One community gave top priority to recruiting medical personnel and facilities. Its supply of physicians, particularly those engaged in general practice, was being depleted through retirement, death, or mobility. New physicians were not moving into the area rapidly enough to meet its medical care needs. Along with efforts to attract physicians, the study committee suggested that, since the citizens in this community paid their share of taxes to support the university medical school, local representatives should confer with officials of the state government in an effort to establish some sort of *quid pro quo* between their tax support for the medical school and the right to expect that a fair proportion of medical students trained by state funds would be returned to their county to practice medicine. The problem was political and financial; it also involved attitudes toward rural practice with which medical education must deal. In addition, this group became involved in a statewide health careers program aimed both at attracting existing health personnel into the area and at recruiting local people into health professions. Within the first year of their program, they experienced some success in recruiting new physicians. In addition, the county commissioners increased the budget for other health personnel. In terms of the entire United States, this study group is small, but in terms of community action to secure needed medical and health personnel, the implications of its work have meaning for hundreds of other communities.

The Cost of a Healthy Community

Health services cost money. Who should provide that money and for which health services are matters of continual debate. Traditionally, the community at large has paid for environmental health services and for the direct personal health services needed by its indigent. Such matters as pure water and sewerage services long ago became part of the common responsibility and were budgeted and financed by tax levies, just as police and fire departments (once staffed only by volunteers) became tax-supported departments in municipalities. But the scope of the health problem has changed, for both environmental and personal service. The effects of one community's actions on another have made it clear that areawide problems cannot be solved solely on the basis of local action. What began as private charity later became primarily publicly financed health services for each community's indigent. This has now become a federally supported program to provide such services for the medically indigent across the nation and insurance for all citizens over 65. At the same time, private prepayment mechanisms have experienced fantastic growth. Furthermore, the taxing structure has changed considerably in recent years; the federal government demands a much larger share in proportion to that received by state and local governments.

It is logical to assume in our expanding economy that more people will be able to pay a larger share of the cost of many of the personal health services they require. Prepaid health plans undoubtedly will continue to provide coverage for an increasing number of these services, either for individuals or for groups of employees whose bargaining with management includes such benefits as part of the employment agreement. However, for years to come, it must be assumed that a large part of the health bill, personal as well as environmental, will be paid by public funds. The present task before the community, then, is that of reaching some agreement, among the towns of a county, the counties of a state, the state itself, and the federal government as to which governmental entity provides what part of the tax dollar for payment of which health costs. These decisions will be rooted in the traditions of every community, as competitors for tax funds state their case at city hall, county courthouse, and state and national capitols.

The costs of health services fall unevenly upon the population; no one can totally predict his need for such services, and his need for them may be entirely unrelated to his ability to pay for them. Because of this unevenness and unpredictability, some form of prepayment is essential. The changing tax structure and the expansion of prepayment programs reflect attempts to find the best way to finance the health services needed in the community. Each makes its own contribution: one provides basic protection; the other, flexibility. Experimentation in combining these two factors should be expected and encouraged as needs change. Fears of governmental control, competition among health-oriented fund-raising groups, and traditional expectations of established facilities must be resolved if communities are to redefine "fair share" in terms of money for health. The hope is that they will be able to do it, through innovation and flexibility.

Every resident of the nation, whether he lives in New York City, the West Virginia hills, the bayous of Louisiana, or the plains, mountain, or coastal areas of the country, should be able to learn about and attain the services necessary for the health of himself, his family, and his neighbors. Communities must make health services available, accessible, and acceptable to all their residents. Our resources include knowledge, wealth, and technology; to those must be added compassion, the willingness to work in concert, agreement on the methods to use, and persistence.

CHAPTER II

Comprehensive Personal Health Services

All communities of this nation must take the action necessary to provide comprehensive personal health services of high quality to all people in each community. These services should embrace those directed toward promotion of positive good health, application of established preventive measures, early detection of disease, prompt and effective treatment, and physical, social, and vocational rehabilitation of those with residual disabilities. This broad range of personal health services must be patterned so as to assure full and intelligent use by all groups in the community.

Success in this endeavor will mean much change. It will require removal of racial, economic, organizational, residence, and geographic barriers to the use of health services. It will require strengthened and expanded licensure and accreditation of services, manpower, and facilities. It will require maximum coverage through health insurance and other prepayment plans, and extension of such insurance to cover the broad range of services both in and out of hospitals. Finally, success will require citizenry that is sufficiently well informed and motivated to follow established principles conducive to good health and to cooperate fully with health services in all phases of prevention and treatment of illness and disability. [B]

The Commission is convinced that comprehensive health services as conceived in its Report can be developed, and must be developed if the full promise of better health is to be realized for all the people. Some communities have taken hold of their health problems and are finding the ways to bring an increasing measure of the potential for better health services to all, and are calling to the full upon the resources of individuals, agencies, and institutions in the process. These are the peaks. Between them are the valleys — communities where poverty, ignorance, prejudice, or lack of resources in people, money, imagination, or initiative still bar the way. There are other valleys where, with all good will, ineptitude or lack of understanding hampers progress.

Addressing itself to this tremendously varied landscape of present services, the Commission sought to identify the concept most basic to a pattern of health services that might lift the heights of the peaks and modify the valleys as they influence the health of the American people today. Communities must look beyond the person who is sick in bed. Each of us needs continuing health services, beginning before birth and lasting throughout our lives. Health services should be brought to bear on the person when he is well, from the moment of birth, and the efforts of that service should be concentrated on keeping him healthy as well as on treating him when ill. This is the concept behind the Commission's use of the word "comprehensive." Communities by deliberate planning must develop patterns of quality comprehensive health services and assure their availability, accessibility, and acceptability to all. This comprehensive approach to health would consider the health needs of all age groups and would offer a full range of services from the promotion of health to rehabilitation after illness. Continuing health education, family planning, the broadest array of safety measures, and all environmental health services appropriate to a given area would be as much a part of such a program as immunization, presymptomatic case finding, and nutritional services. Effective programs for school, mental, industrial, occupational, and dental health would contribute to it. Early diagnosis and treatment of illness and systematic follow-up aimed at restoring the patient to the fullest life possible are basic to this concept.

To make the concept work, the community would need access to a wide range of facilities and services. Besides the hospital and physician's office, the community needs such resources as nursing homes and coordinated home care programs. If, in addition, the community undertakes studies including regular analyses of the patterns of sickness and death in the community, the effectiveness of its health programs, and threats posed by social and environmental changes, it can identify its high-risk groups and develop special programs of consultation and service needed to cope with its health problems. [B-1]

The achievement of goals thus envisioned will call for broad community planning of a type that is just beginning to develop in the United States. The community planning process has been scrutinized by the Commission's Community Action Studies Project; its findings are reflected in this report. Specific health services will vary from community to community as local needs, preferences, customs, and capacities determine, but the range of kinds and quality of services for which all communities can strive are increasingly clear. Many services should be available to the patient in his own home. As needed, they should also be available in physicians' offices, in outpatient clinics, in hospitals, and in facilities for extended care. They should be rounded out by an organized plan for home care for post-hospital patients and for those who do not need hospitalization, by rehabilitative services for the disabled and by mental health services that are fully integrated with all the other services of the community.

Medical care is usually requested and delivered today in an atmosphere of sporadic bursts of concentrated attention, rather than as a continuing, lifelong program of health maintenance. Attitudes toward medical care and traditional concepts of medical practice have created this situation. Changes will be intimately related to the removal of barriers to the use of health services by all persons, to the development of an increasingly well-informed citizenry, and to the extension of health insurance and other prepayment plans, both as to persons covered and range of services covered. The individual frequently may not seek care for a number of reasons. He may fear pain, the unknown, rebuff because of race or economic status, or loss of his identity. He may not know where to find care. It may take too much time or be seriously inconvenient. Or he may not be able to pay for it. Until the problem of paying for regular care is resolved by new and extended methods of financing, costs that must be borne at the time of illness will continue to foster sporadic care of episodes of illness rather than continuous health supervision with emphasis on prevention.

In some instances the mores of medical practice contribute to this care of episodic illness instead of continuous supervision. Overburdened practitioners rarely schedule periodic health evaluation of their patients and follow-up if the evaluation is missed. A large proportion of patients with chronic conditions such as diabetes, hypertension, and nephritis become "lost" from medical supervision because of absence of an organized system of follow-up. The physician must accept the responsibility and take the initiative to assure continuity of care including periodic physical evaluation and preventive and follow-up care. The essentialness of continuity is fully established in fields such as infant care and maternity care, but needs to be extended to cover the entire range of patient care. Physicians would do well to take a leaf from the book of the dentists and send reminders to patients when periodic examinations are due.

The effect on the individual becomes apparent when a man gets sick, and perhaps frightened. With a fire-engine approach, he seeks care, which by that time frequently must be concentrated care in a hospital bed, surrounded by the best available medical talent. Better use of the community's resources would have been achieved if scarce professional skills could have been applied as appropriate to keep the patient from getting sick in the first place.

Sick or well, most people at some time in their lives need one or more of the components of comprehensive health services. Today, the patient often stands a good chance of getting lost in the maze created by the many varied and frequently separate types of services or facilities he may require. Although the job of tying together the separate components of the health system will not be easy, nevertheless, all persons and agencies responsible for health services must foster the gradual building of an integrated program that will provide comprehensive personal health services of optimum quality, equally available and accessible to all, in each community. Separate systems of health care now exist for many groups in the population such as veterans, labor organizations, merchant seamen, and the medically indigent. The welding of separate systems into a community-wide program would preclude new construction or expansion of hospitals for separate population groups. The objective is a gradual integration of such facilities into services for the entire community. [B-2]

Not only is there fragmentation of facilities by ownership or sponsorship, by type of service, and by location, there is also fragmentation among and within the professions, due in large part to specialization. The patient often faces a difficult decision on how to break into the system; once having done so, he may reach a cul-de-sac and drop out, or he may face continuing obstacles in finding his way from one part of it to the other. His entry into the health services pattern may be brought about through the services of a specialist who may interpret his responsibility to be only to refer, not to see that the patient is guided through various facilities and services.

To make it possible for the individual to have easy access to health care, and to facilitate coordinated, continuing health care in a comprehensive services pattern,

every individual should have a personal physician who is the central point for integration and continuity of all medical and medically related services to his patient. Such a physician will emphasize the practice of preventive medicine, through his own efforts and in partnership with the health and social resources of the community.

The physician should be aware of the many and varied social, emotional, and environmental factors that influence the health of his patient and his patient's family. He will either render, or direct the patient to, whatever services best suit his needs. His concern will be for the patient as a whole and his relationship with the patient must be a continuing one. In order to carry out his coordinating role, it is essential that all pertinent health information be channeled through him regardless of what institution, agency, or individual renders the service. He will have knowledge of the access to all health resources of the community — social, preventive, diagnostic, therapeutic, and rehabilitative — and will mobilize them for the patient. [C]

All arrangements for organizing or delivering personal health services should be based on a firm and continuing relationship between the individual patient and a personal physician. This personal physician is responsible for bringing the individual into the integrated program and comprehensive personal health services and for providing or securing needed health care. [C-1]

The concept of the personal physician relates to an approach to the over-all needs of the patient, irrespective of the setting in which he receives health care, and irrespective of the specialty of the physician or the arrangement under which he practices. In itself, this concept places deliberate and necessary emphasis on the fact that all individuals — all families — should have access to a physician who is willing to accept responsibility as the central source for preventive health service and continuing care.

The Commission recognizes the long-range import of this recommendation and its impact on medical manpower and on the institutions that train that manpower; one task force devoted its entire effort to this. Nevertheless, much in the way of current practice and trends supports the Commission's belief that, even in the face of presently increasing percentages of physicians going into specialty practice, there is enough to build upon to span the period of transition required for a substantial reorientation of medical education and the development of adequate numbers of personal physicians. There are now a number of kinds of physicians serving as personal physicians with respect to their patients' over-all health needs. Among them are general practitioners and such specialists as internists, pediatricians, obstetricians, and gynecologists.

It is critically important to make full use of available medical manpower. The physician is neither nurse, social worker, nor physical therapist. He is a physician. His training and talents as a physician must not be dissipated by employing them — except in crisis situations — in any tangential, nonmedical discipline. There are not enough of him in the United States today to warrant wasting a minute of his education and experience on jobs others can do as well. Because it is necessary to face up to this fact squarely, and make the most efficient use of limited physician manpower, health care functions not requiring medical training should be delegated by the physician to other members of the health care team to the maximum extent practical. [C-1]

Theoretically, it is easy enough to stipulate that the personal physician is responsible for seeing his patients through all needed health care services, providing those services within his competence, and making arrangements for additional needed services. However, practical facts of life negate such a theoretical model in its pure form. The patient may become ill in another city, or he may be accidentally injured and rushed to the nearest emergency service. Also, the personal physician is only human and cannot be on constant 24-hour duty; he must sleep, have some recreation, and participate in family and community activities. He himself may become ill, and, if he is to continue to be an effective physician, he will need to devote blocks of time to continuing education.

The nearest approach to the theoretical model would be groups of physicians, large or small, whose arrangements would allow any one of them to serve as personal physician to a patient at any time when that patient's own physician was unavailable. Such functional arrangements should be on a regular, continuing basis, and inherent responsibilities would need to be understood and accepted by the physicians involved. Patients too would need to understand and accept these arrangements, which should go into effect at any time the personal physician is "de facto" unavailable. To fulfill his role as "backstop" for the personal physician, his associate would need access to medical records sufficiently complete to enable him to substitute effectively. The personal physician should therefore maintain an established relationship with other physicians in order to make medical service available to his patient at all times, 24 hours a day, seven days a week. The need for such back-up is as important for the patient who receives medical care from a physician practicing as an individual as for the patient of a physician who is part of an organized group.

Organizational arrangements, ranging from informal associations to formally organized groups, merit exploration as a means toward integrating personal health services in a community. Emphasis should be on forms of associations among physicians that would maintain high standards of care, correct undesirable fragmentation of health services by bringing many specialists and specialized services into proximity, and facilitate payment mechanisms that reduce economic barriers to preventive services and prompt diagnostic and therapeutic services. [C-3]

Between the extremes of solo practice and formal group practice, there is great promise in the concept of a physicians' office building providing for shared common facilities and involving proven referral patterns. Where feasible, such a building should be located adjacent to a hospital. If the official health agency is nearby, the possibility for comprehensive community health services is strengthened.

Communications systems should be organized to give the personal physician ready access to the total medical history of his patient at any given point in time. Present record keeping compromises both quality and economy of health care, and reflects fragmentation by administering agency, type of service, and location.

Group practice of medicine, as a specific way of integrating the services of physicians, has demonstrated that it can provide an effective and efficient method of furnishing comprehensive medical care of good quality. Such organization of services should be stimulated and encouraged as one of the best routes toward comprehensive personal health services with the understanding that for each patient, one physician is his personal physician. [C-3] Group practices require the services of nurses, social workers, laboratory technicians, receptionists, accountants, and other allied personnel. Therefore, the model for provision of health care has grown from the individual, his family, his personal physician and associates, to include a number of additional persons and services. Such groups are in operation in many parts of the country. However, the potential contribution to their effectiveness of a full use of visiting nurses, organized programs of home care, medical social workers, physical therapists, clinical psychologists, and other professional associates working on a regular basis with personal physicians as an integral part of the organization should be further developed.

Although the personal physician can provide a great deal of health care in his office or his patient's home, certain diagnostic and treatment services can best be provided in a hospital. Every hospital should have a service for personal physicians, and, conversely, every qualified personal physician should have a staff appointment in one or more accredited hospitals with privileges in accordance with his capabilities. Each personal physician should also have access to a program of continuing medical education.

The personal physician should have available to him and should utilize the full range of community health services, within and outside the hospital. He will be working with a team in which the special abilities of the different members are integrated for a common purpose — the health and well-being of the patient. Many of these skills have been available to him in the hospital and other institutions in the past and more will be needed in the future. Now there is an urgent need to find ways for him to use these talents and skills in the home and in connection with other outpatient services. The medical profession should accentuate its work with community leaders to develop means through which this can be accomplished. [C-2] If the personal physician is to mobilize all applicable community resources for the benefit of his patients, he will need to learn more about them himself, use the assistance of public health nurses and social workers in health departments, hospitals, and welfare agencies, and utilize Health Service Information and Referral centers where they are available.

To some physicians, especially recent graduates of medical schools that include within their curricula effective courses on community medicine, this is a fascinating and challenging medical world. But to far more, it is a world with many unknowns, which calls for a type of practice for which numerous experienced and successful physicians have not been prepared. The medical world they know appears safe and secure in comparison with the road leading toward comprehensive health services. Fortunately, many physicians are challenged by the medical frontiers they can see emerging for preventive medicine practiced in a community setting in partnership with other health personnel. In such a program, the physician can intervene at a time and place, prior to medical crisis, to keep his patient in good health as well as to treat him when he is ill. He will apply his knowledge of prevention every time he diagnoses and treats a patient, will be watching in the home, his office, or medical facility for opportunities to bring that knowledge into practice, and will repeat his preventive techniques as often and for as long as necessary to protect the health of families under his care.

Recruiting and Educating Physicians
for Comprehensive Health Care

The Commission recommends that a start be made now to produce the needed number and quality of personal physicians for the delivery of comprehensive personal health services in the decades ahead. This will require a nationwide effort to provide appropriate educational opportunities and career incentives, taking into account the established framework of specialization. Attracting the medical graduate to a career as a personal physician will be possible only if there is general recognition of the importance of his role and he is accorded status, professional satisfaction, and income comparable to that of other physicians. The program required to produce these personal physicians will be comparable in magnitude to that which expanded medical research in the past two decades. Large-scale financing will be necessary for support of teachers, trainees, facilities, programs, and educational research.

Medical schools will have to alter very considerably their present intramural curriculum and develop community-based and community-oriented teaching programs as part of the training experience. Universities presenting medical education should provide a continuum of experience: premedical, medical, internship, residency, and continuing education.

To educate personal physicians and attract the interest of medical students to careers in this area, programs which emphasize the continuity of relationship between the physician and the patient, and the responsibility of the physician for assuring comprehensive care, must be developed. The personal physician of the future must have a broader knowledge of all the elements of comprehensive health services than he now receives during his training — graduate and undergraduate. His clinical education and residency program should place emphasis on the development of basic competence in preventive medicine, internal medicine, pediatrics, psychiatry, and rehabilitation. The American Medical Association and the Association of American Medical Colleges should take the initiative in developing specific recommendations to universities for the undergraduate and graduate training of personal physicians. Further, university medical centers should accept the responsibility for providing personal health services to a limited but representative sample of the population through a demonstration unit designed for teaching and research on comprehensive health care. The training of specialists will and should continue, but the education of all physicians should include appropriate courses and experience in community medicine.

Means should be found to secure status for the personal physician and income comparable to that of other specialists, and the medical profession should give serious consideration to according him status by the establishment of an appropriate board certification.

In view of the complexity of medical knowledge and the speed of change, medical schools should take the initiative in developing programs of continuing education with the cooperation of other groups such as the medical society, hospitals, and health departments. [C-4] Sharp focus should be given now to preparing internists, general practitioners, pediatricians, and others who, for the foreseeable future, will in part have to play the role of the personal physician, especially in solo practice situations.

Training for comprehensive health care may continue to be in medical centers or it may be necessary to establish new kinds of teaching centers, but one thing is certain: training for personal physicians, as much as for surgeons, pediatricians, or any other physicians, must be based directly on student experience with actual patients and it must convey to the student knowledge of community living situations. He should learn about a community while he learns about medicine.

Of course the patient must also be educated. Appropriate health institutions and professions should make a concerted effort to teach the public the desirability of selecting a personal physician and the importance of frequent contact with him.

Tackling Special Problems

Comprehensive health services should help to resolve some special problems that technically are controllable but which are not being successfully coped with. Much disease and illness can be prevented through early detection techniques. Many disabilities need not occur, or could be substantially corrected. Infant mortality rates can be reduced. These problems and many others, including less tangible ones of health education and motivation, should respond favorably to the forces of continuity and coordination of services inherent in the concept of comprehensive personal health services. From the time the individual comes in contact with the system, he should be encouraged to increase his understanding and sense of responsibility for maintaining his own health.

One special problem is cancer of the lung, which could be dramatically reduced if people would stop smoking cigarettes. In competition with multi-million-dollar advertising, relatively little effort has been made to stress the hazards of smoking. There is, however, evidence of some effectiveness with young people. Such efforts should be accelerated. Research must provide insight into ways to make smoking socially unacceptable at the same time it seeks other solutions. In general, it is true that with present medical knowledge hundreds of thousands of lives a year could be saved if we applied techniques fully and if they were acted on. For example, heart disease and stroke are indubitably related to an individual's way of life, and their toll could be reduced by broader observance of well-established guidelines of exercise, diet, and weight control.

Social pressure, social habits, conflicting values, fear, or other nonmedical factors may complicate health problems so that medicine in its traditional sense cannot solve them alone. Some can be met by general social advance. We know that there is a relation between poverty and short life expectancy. The community health team must coordinate its work with efforts aimed at the eradication of poverty; in this, as in other difficult problems, it must join in educating the public and in planning which extends beyond the limits of health facilities and services.

Accessibility and Acceptability

Unfortunately, it is not enough to provide health services that are accessible; they must be used by the people who need them. How can residents of a community be taught to make proper use of existing services? How can facilities and personnel be assembled so that they are easily available and reasonably priced?

Medical services and facilities in many communities seem to be situated more for the convenience of the health personnel than for the consumer of health services. Old people and women with small children who have to change buses to get care, and who cannot afford taxis, become discouraged. Many have neither the time nor the strength to seek treatment if it means traveling to several facilities or if office hours do not coincide with times at which a man can leave his job or a mother her children.

Obtaining community-based health care must be made quicker, easier, and less painful. Rescheduling of practices in the health field can benefit both those who provide the services and those who use them. If the patient's waiting time is cut down, and if the shuffling of patients among medical units can be decreased, patients will be more receptive to medical care. Evening hours for preventive and therapeutic services could alleviate problems for many and stimulate greater use of those services.

There is little reason to believe that communities generally will or should break with our pluralistic traditions. Not every community will achieve the same ends through the same means, and the Commission accepts the desirability of these differences in molding a community pattern which will bring all health services into a comprehensive system. Whatever the pattern, it should include in each community an effective counseling, placement, and referral service for patients in cooperation with the health care facilities system and the professions providing health services. [B-3]

Consistent high quality of health care is essential, and every community must bear the responsibility for accepting only one standard: the best health care it can give for all people. It must insist that the places in which its health services are provided meet criteria established by regulatory and accrediting agencies outside of the community.

While much has been done to provide communities with standards of high quality care on which they can in confidence rely, much remains to be done. Among others, the Joint Commission on Accreditation of Hospitals, the American Public Health Association, and the National League for Nursing have lighted many paths to good performance by providers of health services. Despite their salutary efforts, some dark passages still exist. They too could be lighted if existing licensing and accreditation procedures for health care facilities and services were strengthened, expanded, and enforced by appropriate authorities. Accreditation should be extended to include nursing homes, rehabilitation facilities, and noninstitutional services such as home nursing and home care. Hospitals and other institutions and facilities and noninstitutional services need to strengthen programs to assure that accreditation standards are met by continuing assessment of performance. [B-5]

The areas of organized home care, rehabilitation, care of the mentally ill, and dentistry are here singled out because the Commission feels the need to stress their relation to the composite of comprehensive personal health services. The time is ripe for these special components to become integrated with the whole. Acting on opportunities provided through legislation and programs of voluntary and professional groups, communities can now take the initiative to assure the availability of these services for their residents.

Organized Home Care Services

For some communities, the steps involved in making comprehensive personal health services available will be primarily those of regrouping and new use of facilities and personnel through cooperative planning; for other communities, they will involve initiating additional services. Most communities have a long distance to go in developing an over-all plan that will ensure the availability of a variety of services appropriate to the patient's needs outside the hospital. These services range from preventive, diagnostic, therapeutic, and rehabilitative services that can be rendered in an outpatient setting, to services needed in a nursing home and programs of care in the patient's own home.

Hospitals and other health agencies must cooperate in the strengthening and development of facilities and services for patients who do not require hospitalization (such as outpatient services, extended care facilities, home care programs, geriatric day centers, and foster family programs) to promote comprehensive personal health care through a network of appropriate alternative settings. [B-6]

Organized home care has long been cited as a greatly needed program for patients requiring extended care and has been highly recommended by groups in the medical, hospital, and public health fields. Provisions for paying for organized home health care for the aged through Social Security should make it possible for many communities to develop such programs. Most communities do not now have them, and programs that do exist serve only a few patients. Many patients in general hospitals, in chronic disease facilities, or in nursing homes could be equally well or better cared for at home if organized home care programs were available.

Good home care programs operate through a centrally administered team approach under medical direction. To be sure that he receives continued care appropriate to his needs, someone must identify the patient, assess his needs on a 24-hour basis, determine the adequacy of the home, and plan accordingly. Such an assessment requires the combined skills of the physician, the public health nurse, and the social worker — all members of the team most familiar with the patient's problems.

Home care, when the situation permits, is more acceptable to many patients, especially the elderly, than institutional care. It has special application to rehabilitation and to care of the mentally ill, as well as to other chronically ill patients. Through such a program, the community can expand, extend, and deliver its health services in a manner acceptable to both the patient and the professional.

Rehabilitation

As a part of the broad spectrum of comprehensive personal health services, rehabilitation cannot be compartmentalized. It blends imperceptibly with prevention, early detection, and treatment of disease. Rehabilitation is concerned with handicap as it affects all ages and occupational groups, and with physical, emotional, and intellectual disability. Just as the personal physician is concerned with prevention of illness, so those working in the field of rehabilitation are concerned with the prevention of handicaps.

No line can or should be drawn between treatment and rehabilitation. The early treatment of ear infections reduces the number and severity of hearing handicaps. Effective medical management of diabetes reduces the number of amputations due to diabetic gangrene. The selection of the amputation site by the surgeon may affect the later efficiency of an artificial limb and the job its wearer may fill.

The concept includes both attitude and technology. In attitude it looks beyond the cure of illness or recovery from accident to planning for all the steps necessary for the patient's full return to normal functioning. The rehabilitation-minded physician does not regard his job as complete when the temperature has returned to normal or when the surgical scar has healed. Success in rehabilitation depends to a large extent on the timing of specific rehabilitation measures. The stroke patient has a much greater potential for functional recovery if rehabilitation techniques are begun within a few days of the stroke rather than months later when the condition may be complicated by contractures, bed sores, and psychological deterioration.

Less than two decades ago, medicine recognized rehabilitation as a specialty by establishing the American Board of Physical Medicine and Rehabilitation. Specialists in this field have developed an ever-widening array of specific techniques and physical devices that aid the rehabilitation process. The patient who is severely disabled or who has multiple disabilities will frequently require extensive services in a rehabilitation center under the direction of a specialist in rehabilitation. However, by its very nature rehabilitation involves all members of the health care team. The cardiac surgeon is a member of that team when he implants a plastic heart valve to replace a diseased one as is the psychiatrist when the patient's emotional reaction to physical handicap becomes a problem. Dentists, social workers, nurses, physical, speech, and occupational therapists, and psychologists all play important roles in rehabilitation.

Rehabilitation reaches beyond the spectrum of health care to include the testing and evaluation of work competence, training for new vocations for which the disability will not be a handicap, and special modification of home, transportation, and place of work to circumvent the disability. The rehabilitation counselor works in these areas and, in collaboration with the health professions, helps guide the patient back to a productive and rewarding place in society.

The Joint Commission on Undergraduate Medical Education in Physical Medicine and Rehabilitation has been engaged in a study of teaching physical medicine and rehabilitation to medical students. Its findings will undoubtedly lead to expansion of the curriculum in more medical schools. Increased emphasis on physical medicine and rehabilitation is needed not only in medical school curriculums, but in internship and residency programs, and in postgraduate medical education programs. Such teaching would provide communities with physicians sensitive to the rehabilitation needs and potential of their patients and technically competent to deal with them. Additional plans must be developed and funds provided to train health personnel other than medical students in all areas of rehabilitation.

Rehabilitation of the severely handicapped has been slowed by the cost, which is nearly always higher than the average family can afford. The patient's family resources and his insurance benefits have usually been exhausted long before the patient is well. The acute phase of his illness or injury is likely to be brief in comparison with the months, or even years, required for rehabilitation. Third parties who provide insurance coverage for medical costs of rehabilitation seldom pay for the expensive equipment and apparatus needed by the disabled person. Hence, new approaches to this problem are indicated. Experiments and demonstrations aimed at providing prepayment coverage as the principal way of making rehabilitation services available to all who need them are of the utmost importance. It is the responsibility of the community to make rehabilitation service available. It is the responsibility of the physician, whatever his special field of interest, to make full use of these services. [B-7]

Comprehensive Community Mental Health Services

Mental health services, too, have been considered as special services in the past. Today, a dynamic, new approach to community-based prevention, treatment, and control of emotional disturbance and mental illness is bringing this specialty back into the mainstream of health services. New mental health programs project hope for emotionally disturbed persons that is more promising than anything that has occurred in treatment of mental illness since man first tried to exorcise evil spirits.

An increasingly urbanized and complex society has produced its own stress patterns. These call for special psychologic and psychiatric measures in connection with health promotion and health care. The application of psychological and social sciences to health deserve increasing recognition by the health professions. The importance of environmental stress in causation and of environmental support in treatment of psychiatric disorders should be recognized in the organization of general medical, occupational, social, and welfare services. Psychiatric services are needed to a varying degree by an appreciable part of those seeking medical care and should be an integral part of all treatment programs. In addition, the current national movement toward comprehensive community mental health and retardation services and the great resources in public interest, experience, and money that have been developed should be integrated into community plans for comprehensive health services. [B-8]

The need to improve and coordinate services for the mentally ill was dramatically demonstrated in the United States during World War II, when, by 1945, 1,091,000 men were rejected by the armed forces as unfit for military service because of neuropsychiatric conditions. Public interest was further aroused by discovery in the 1950's of the first effective psychoactive drugs, the tranquilizers and antidepressants, and also by persistent efforts on the part of citizens' groups to obtain better treatment for the mentally ill and mentally retarded in state mental hospitals and custodial institutions.

Following publication in 1961 of the report of the Joint Commission on Mental Illness and Health, *Action for Mental Health*, federal funds have stimulated the assessment of the mental health resources and needs of each state and the construction and initial staffing of community mental health centers.

The modern concept behind the program to provide preventive and treatment services is that most persons suffering from emotional and mental disorders can best be treated in their home communities, rather than in isolated hospitals. Quality treatment should be designed to provide a continuity of care for the individual patient, adapted to his needs, so that he can return quickly to a productive life, given rehabilitation and aftercare to control any residual disability.

The Commission believes that the traditional separation of physical and mental illness, promoted by the existence of separate treatment systems, is outmoded and harmful. Communities need to look at treatment of the man whose mind is sick in the same way they consider treatment of the primarily physical disorders. In 1965, psychiatric patients were admitted for diagnosis and treatment to more than 1000 general hospitals. Community mental health centers will make it possible for personal physicians to participate in the psychiatric treatment of their patients and to maintain the continuity of care that is the modern health objective.

Destined for years past to be locked up indefinitely in state mental hospitals, the mentally ill will, more and more, be treated in their home communities. Medical schools are adding community psychiatry to the curriculum of their departments of psychiatry in increasing numbers, and funds are available to train physicians in short courses in psychiatry, so that all medical practitioners will be able to treat the less severe disturbances and to diagnose the need for special psychiatric treatment.

Unified Dental Health Program   **1511357**

One-fourth of our children have teeth and jaws that are so poorly aligned that the children are handicapped by facial disfigurement or inability to chew properly. Oral clefts — cleft palates — are second only to clubfoot as the most common birth defect and account for 13 percent of birth defects. One of every 40 cancer deaths — 5000 a year — is caused by oral cancer. Almost half our people aged 55 or over have lost all their teeth. The potential dividends of an organized, comprehensive community program of dental health services are great if that program includes prevention, early diagnosis and treatment, regular maintenance, and continuous efforts to educate the public.

Among available preventive procedures, fluoridation of drinking water is remarkable for its simplicity of application and its

effectiveness in reducing tooth decay by two-thirds. Nevertheless, during the first 15 years that this preventive was available,
only 3,000 communities with a population of 60,000,000 adopted
it. The Commission strongly supports fluoridation in every community in the nation.

Tooth decay and most gum diseases are not self-healing; they
become progressively more severe and complicated when treatment is neglected or postponed. Treatment thus becomes complex, costly, and wasteful of the community's dental facilities
and manpower.

Organized efforts in communities will be necessary if our children are to be guaranteed a good chance for dental health. A
nation of such communities is in accord with the 1965 resolution
of the American Dental Association directing its Council on
Dental Health and other agencies of the Association to "develop
a national program for children, particularly the needy and un-
derprivileged, in order to make the benefits of modern dental
health service available to all children of the nation."

In 1965, the American people spent a relatively large proportion of their total expenditures for health care on dental health
services — approximately ten cents out of every dollar. If these
funds could be spent for appropriately timed preventive services,
for incremental or maintenance treatment services, and for effective education of the public, great strides would be made toward
the attainable goal of lifetime teeth for all.

Administrative Research

Community action to make comprehensive personal health
services available will undoubtedly result in better health for
that community's people, but it will require more of the community than simply adapting to a blueprint. The ever-changing
health scene cannot be reduced to a filled-in plan, drawn in advance. Much will depend on the vision and experimentation put
to work within each community.

In their task communities need the backing of stepped-up
investment in administrative research on how to deliver health
services in the community. There is universal endorsement of
and support for the scientific search for greater knowledge of
the causes, treatment, and prevention of disease and illness. Re-

search into improved methods of delivery needs the same kind of endorsement and support. Administrative research in applying scientific knowledge has been grossly neglected; it lags far behind our developing of that scientific knowledge. The need is urgent. There should be increased research and demonstration to develop improved methods of organization and delivery of health services and to improve the quality of such services. [B-9]

Between the methods of health administration and the objectives they are designed to achieve, there exists a relationship which has not yet been closely enough scrutinized. Research into the organization and delivery of health services constitutes one of the most important and forward-looking steps toward the goal of comprehensive personal health services for all.

CHAPTER III

Comprehensive Environmental Health Services

The quality of living has been strained in this country. The gentle rain from heaven as it drops upon the earth beneath is also likely to drop Strontium 90 on the vegetation. Thoughtful members of the health professions, with others, are aware of this, and much of today's questioning revolves around the means, the methods, and the ways to secure for ourselves and our posterity a quality of life commensurate with the quality of our knowledge *about* the good life.

Environmental health programs can make a positive contribution to people's health and well-being.

Optimum health can be fostered by prospective planning and management of comprehensive environmental health services. This means going far beyond assuring pure water, clean air, and safe food. It means assuring hygienic housing to provide space for adequate privacy and family sociability, for places of rest and quiet and places for activity and recreation. It means assuring an external milieu for man designed to stimulate his greatest growth potential. [D]

All of this can be encompassed in the word "environment" — each person's room for living. For some, this means warmth and security, coupled with excitement, thought, achievement, and rewards. For others, the meaning of the word "environment" is communicated through the angry, frightened, or tortured questions: "Where am I? How did I get here? How can I get out?"

People in the health professions are today faced with a problem that faces all questioning minds. There is basic empiricism; there is clinical experiment. Where do they begin and end? The new awareness of the complexities of our environment and their effects upon our health compel re-examination. The sciences of tissues and organisms must be examined in the light of our growing knowledge of behavior and subjective experience. The crisis of environment is upon us.

The American environment is being contaminated at a rate rapidly approaching saturation and the health of the people is in jeopardy. The need for decisive citizen action is urgent. Moreover, people are using physical, biological, and chemical products indiscriminately, unaware, for the most part, of their hazards.

Improving the quality of our environment requires additional financial resources, public and private, adequately planned and programmed to insure the control of water and air pollution and protective measures against contamination from physical, biological, and chemical products, including the increasing use of radioactive materials. [E]

Air, water, and land are not unlimited and the maintenance of these resources at high quality becomes daily a more complicated challenge to all leadership — political, governmental, industrial, business, labor, educational, and agricultural.

In the past, most public health professionals looked upon the environment of the community to which they were responsible as a series of interlocking, but nevertheless quite clean-cut, situations to be controlled by application of specific methods to particular situations. While environmental specialists have recognized the broad concept inherent in the word "environment," they have conceived of their mission in a more narrow sense, namely the physical, chemical, and nonhuman biologic forces that surround man. The usual understanding of the term "environment," as currently employed in public health thinking and practice, has excluded man as a component of the environment except to the extent that he alters its physical, chemical, and nonhuman biologic character.

The Commission believes that this concept is valid as far as it goes, but that it does not go far enough. Man himself must be further studied to learn more about why he behaves as he does. In attempting to meet the modern hazards of the environment, health departments and health officers must be joined by behavioral scientists, among others, if this nation is to reverse the trend toward an unlivable environment.

Acceptable health care for the individual cannot be provided in a contaminated environment. In this nuclear day, citizen understanding of adequate health care must make a quantum jump forward to acceptance of a tenet long advocated by alert public health agencies: that personal and environmental health are inseparable. All public health agencies must assert strong leadership in attaining a safe environment; they have an inescapable responsibility for maintaining a safe environment. Because of that responsibility, public health agencies should administer those programs where the protection and promotion of health is the primary objective. Where health is not the primary objective and a program is administered by another agency, the public health agency should have responsibility for establishing and assuring enforcement of environmental health standards. [E-1]

Public health agencies, in presenting new concepts, more effective methodology, and better processes for working with others, must accept a shared responsibility with industry, commerce, and agriculture, and with the consumer interests of the community itself for participation in all aspects of program planning, operation, and evaluation of environmental health. No longer, in evolving and enforcing effective controls on man to save his environment, can the health agency project plans based on traditional patterns. The time has come when man, having almost ruined certain aspects of his environment, must use his mind, his money, and his muscle to keep the environment from ruining him.

There is no longer any lack of realization that the environment is a totality; that its impact on the human being is the effect of the sum total of all contaminants, acting separately or in concert. Even when people do not fully understand the precise health implications of a particular group of contaminants they know that pollution is an undesirable and detrimental factor in their lives, that it should be eliminated, and that to do this will take money. In our efforts to abate pollution we are farther ahead in some programs than in others. Where progress is lagging it will be necessary to accentuate research and program development to deal with the rapidly escalating pollution hazards.

By 1965, we had begun to understand the kinds of research necessary to attack our environmental problems. From 1961 to 1966, at least three major committees of eminent scientists issued lengthy reports; at least seven major books dealing with the general problem and its importance appeared on the market. During the same four years the United States Public Health Service expanded its activities in environmental health. It established new organizations to work on problems of solid waste and on the health effects of pesticides. Many other parts of the health establishment, such as, for example, the National Cancer Institute, were studying specific aspects of environmental contamination. The National Environmental Health Sciences Center has been established to conduct research necessary to understand the long-term biological effects of the environment on man, and to maintain the overview of our national effort in this field. It was also charged with the responsibility to identify emerging problems and to coordinate a complete national research program. While this basic research is underway, research in each categorical field must be continued and made more effective. Research required in air and water pollution, radiological health, and occupational and industrial health must be intensified and must be supported by organized reporting of disease (as well as death) caused by or related to environmental pollutants.

Two percent of the pool of scientific manpower was engaged in environmental health work in 1965, and the estimate for 1970 is that 2.6 percent will be so employed. Most of this small fraction of the whole body of scientists is involved in seeking solutions to the largest fraction of the total environmental problem — air, water, and food pollution. It may be well to look at these essential constituents of life and their impact on community environment — for good when they are clean, for evil when they are contaminated. We will look very briefly, as well, at solid waste disposal, radiation hazards, occupational health, and also at injuries caused by accidents. It is recognized that, although these seven are representative of the environmental health problem, there are many others hardly less critical. A more detailed discussion of the broad range of environmental hazards and health consideration is contained in the report of the Commission's Task Force on Environmental Health.

Air and Water Pollution

The problems of air and water pollution are often linked, and they do have much in common; but there is one basic difference. It is still possible for man to purify water that has been contaminated, but we do not know how to purify air for all the people just before they breathe it. People are in the same relative position with regard to air pollution as are fish with regard to water pollution.

The basic problem is caused by the following facts of modern life. People and sources of pollution tend to concentrate in the same places. Pollution is caused when we transport ourselves or our goods and services from one place to another. Population concentrations coincident with industrial, municipal, and domestic activities add startling amounts of gaseous and solid pollutants to both air and water, and, as our technological and scientific knowledge widens, new kinds of pollutants are added to the old. For example, pollutants come from the combustion of fuels for heat and power, from industrial processing, from the disposal of waste by burning, and from the imperfect combustion of motor vehicle fuels, among many sources. And, while these sources continue to increase, the supply of air and water into which pollution goes remains constant.

In the nineteenth century, a few cities began air pollution programs primarily because the obvious pollutant — smoke — was dirty. Today, however, many of the more serious pollutants are invisible gases. We are increasingly concerned about the health effects of the ordinary level of air pollution to which city dwellers are exposed during much of their lifetime. Long-term exposure to air pollution has been associated with lung cancer and with many chronic respiratory diseases, such as asthma, bronchitis, and emphysema. Evidence that air pollution is a factor in chronic respiratory disease continues to accumulate. How, then, can air pollution control be effected?

The problem cannot be solved by any community alone. Air moves across county and continent and it carries its pollutants with it. Effective control programs must be based on the air pollution "community of solution." Since air movements do not respect political lines, the remedial programs cannot be restricted by local or state political jurisdictions. The air pollution communities of solution will be large and will coincide closely with industrial centers. A beginning has been made by establishing air pollution monitoring stations in specific areas of the United States. The size of the problem dictates a nationwide, continuous, automated air sampling network that will include every community that is a potential or known source of air pollution, whether that pollution be biological, chemical, or radiological. Such sampling would provide a basis for the development of prevention and control programs in communities. [E-2]

Governmental and industrial funds must be provided in vastly increased amounts to assist in developing adequate research and control programs, but the prevention and elimination of sources of pollution must proceed on the basis of present knowledge. [E-3]

It is no longer necessary to prove that our air is becoming increasingly polluted; we all know it from personal experience. We also know that the rate of air pollution is increasing and will continue to increase unless decisive control measures are put into effect promptly. The provisions of the Clean Air Act and the 1965 amendments, if put into general practice and vigilantly enforced, will represent a good beginning. The Clean Air Act places greater responsibility for control on state and local communities and makes federal funds available to assist them. It also gives the federal government power to take action to abate air pollution problems beyond the control of individual communities. Additionally, the Secretary of the Department of Health, Education, and Welfare can initiate abatement procedures when pollution arising in one state is adversely affecting the health or welfare of persons in another state. The 1965 amendment gives him authority to establish and enforce standards on the pollutional discharges of new motor vehicles by September 1, 1967. Many persons are concerned that even this time schedule is inadequate, but it has the advantage of securing the maximum research efforts on the part of the automotive, oil, and other industries to devise effective control mechanisms, cleaner fuel, and more efficient motors.

Legislation is not the whole answer, however. Even though federal legislation now gives special emphasis to sulphur emissions from coal and oil burning and to automobile exhaust, we still do not know how to control them adequately; this will require more research, and that research must be done by industry, universities, and health departments aided by federal and foundation grant support. Industry must increase its effort to find a means of power for automobiles and trucks that will minimize their contribution to the air pollution problem. Meanwhile, the federal government should exercise its interstate commerce powers to encourage manufacturers to continue voluntary efforts to improve currently available devices that reduce health hazards from pollution. The federal government, in cooperation with state health and motor vehicle agencies, should require that all motor vehicles be equipped with the most effective means of eliminating the noxious gases from motor exhausts. [E-4]

Public concern, evidenced both in news media and in legislation, is beginning to provide the public health officer with an attentive audience for his concern over correction of public health hazards. The National Water Quality Act, for example, provides that states must promulgate adequate water quality standards by June 1967; if they do not, the federal government will. Representatives of the major industries differ in their approaches to the problem. Some say that the cleanup demands are unrealistically rigorous and costly; others, that the demands are being met; and others, that industry must unite to meet them, perhaps helped by federal subsidy. But whatever the attitude, the fact is that water pollution in this country has become so widespread that a federal statute has been enacted to force improvement.

Basic to the solution of pollution of our streams, rivers, and lakes — not to mention the backyard wells that supply many a septic-tanked suburbia — is an adequate answer to the sewage disposal question. The nation must increase the power of its attack on water pollution. An unprecedented, large-scale effort is required to develop and finance comprehensive water pollution control programs. As part of such programs, the existing ceiling for the federal sewage treatment facilities grant program should be eliminated. If we regard sewerage systems as a national resource, it will lead to consideration of a different method of financing their construction and maintenance, somewhat analogous to that currently used for interstate highway systems, with federal sources financing the major portion of the system, and state and local sources supplying sewer lines as necessary to tie into the main system. At the same time, research efforts to find new methods of sewage disposal or conversion must continue. [E-5]

Food Protection

Although the true incidence of food-borne illness is unknown, because of grossly incomplete reporting, estimates put the number of such illnesses, occurring annually in the United States, at over a million cases, and recent epidemiological information indicates this incidence may be on the rise.

The current level of support being given to food protection at all levels of government is grossly inadequate. It does not even permit the responsible agencies to apply available knowledge to prevent such illnesses, much less to cope with the multitude of new and emerging problems. In fact, there is an enormous and rapidly increasing disparity between the number of problems arising and the amount of effort directed to their resolution. Changes in the production and processing of foods, increasing exposure of foods to chemicals, and changes in food preparation and nationwide distribution methods and techniques, together with inadequate public health controls, have created the potential for massive nationwide outbreaks of food-borne illnesses.

To meet these challenges there is an urgent need for increased research and investigation to identify and evaluate the public health implications of changes and developments occurring in all segments of a dynamic food industry. Equally important is the need for resources, facilities, and training to assure translation of available and newly developed knowledge into food protection practices which are practical of application on a day-to-day basis by the more than 4,000,000 persons working in the industry.

Solid Waste Disposal

Disposing of solid wastes, or converting them to other uses, often contributes to both air and water pollution. From smoldering dumps to water-dumped sludge the pollution spreads. To deal with the fast-growing problems of solid waste disposal, that disposal must be planned and operated on a problem-shed basis. Health agencies must establish community standards for collecting and disposing of solid wastes and, in cooperation with other responsible operating agencies, exercise leadership in evaluating the adequacy of these activities. State governments must adopt enabling legislation to provide their political subdivisions with workable legal and administrative tools to perform this function effectively. Research must be unremitting. Industry, foundations, voluntary agencies, and government must recognize the high priority of efforts to cope with the mountains of waste that are the discards from our civilization. [E-6]

Our country has become too small to accommodate the indiscriminate disposal of its unwanted by-products. There is little reason to doubt that the ingenuity and skill which has built our nation's productivity can be successfully put to work to solve the problems that very productivity spawns. Industry needs to recognize that the cost of waste treatment is a legitimate part of the cost of its products. It should be required to reduce its contribution to the pollution of both air and water. [E-7]

But industry, its factories, and automobiles are not the only contributors to the problem. Communities themselves are at fault, when they fail to handle their sewage and waste disposal problems adequately, as are government installations, which often are guilty of contributing to the problem. As a first step toward cleaner air and water, all federal, state, and local institutions must end their own contribution to pollution. [E-8]

Every conceivable sector, segment, and individual in the United States is in some way responsible for pollution, and must be made aware of this. Although effective control cannot be achieved by one local community, neither can it be achieved nationally until there is broad public understanding of the problem and enlightened community leadership to solve it. Effective control programs will be established as soon as the people understand sufficiently the need to insist on corrective action — not before.

In Los Angeles, for example, the air pollution problem was so evident to every resident that the public supported an effective control program. Los Angeles still has smog — mainly because we do not yet know how to capture some of the gaseous pollutants or change them chemically into nontoxic forms — but that city's air pollution control system is the most outstanding one in the world, and has undoubtedly made the continued growth of the city possible. Similar systems for both air and water must be developed in many more areas, and the hour is late.

Occupational Health

The occupational health problem of the nation is in need of a major attack. We must seek to eliminate any factor which may make a worker pay with his health or his life for the privilege of having a job. We cannot afford the lowered production that results from correctable health factors associated with the place of work. We must make arrangements to cope with the occupational health problems of workers in small plants, where most of our workers are employed, so that they have health protection on the job similar to that provided in modern larger plants.

Radiation Hazards

Radiation hazards stem from the pollution of the environment by radioactive materials from industrial use and from medical use of X rays and radioactive materials. Although the major exposure to ionizing radiation is in the diagnostic and therapeutic use of X rays and radioactive agents, the hazards of exposure from air, water, food, and industrial sources also require attention. Advancing technology has not only carried along with it dangers to health in contaminated air and water, it has introduced another and more sophisticated evil — the hazard of overdoses of radiation, whether borne by air, water, or food or resulting from industrial exposure. Debate about the precise amount of ionizing radiation a human being can absorb without danger must not interrupt programs designed to control the hazard.

Some radiation hazards defy geographic containment. Local communities may be able to establish effective control standards for radiological hazards arising from X-ray use, but radioactive wastes polluting waterways ignore political boundaries and may become serious state and interstate problems. The hazards of radiological pollution are global in dimension, and enlightened nations are seeking to control them. Meanwhile, the concept of comprehensive community health services requires that citizens recognize the existence of the problem in their plans to improve health care in their own communities. If it is an international problem, it is no less an intercommunity problem, best managed, because of its sweeping nature, by state health departments with strong support from the federal government — but with the ultimate solution to be found through international agreement on the release of radioactive materials into the environment.

Preventing Accidents

Accidents are the fourth leading cause of death in the nation; in children, teenagers, and young adults, they are the leading cause. At any given time there are 11,000,000 persons suffering from some chronic defect or impairment resulting from accidental injury; 38 percent of all noninstitutionalized impairments are due to accidental injury. Much of this toll of injury and death can be prevented by the application of currently available techniques. When accidents do occur, then the task is to minimize their ill effects by prompt and adequate medical attention, from first aid through to rehabilitation. The mobilization of community health resources should be directed toward these goals.

In general, most accidents are caused by factors present at the time and scene of the accident. Underlying factors, mostly behavioral, although not so evident at the time, are also important.

There was a time in this country when winding dirt roads and two-lane concrete highways patched with tar crossed the metal tracks of the Iron Horse; underpasses, overpasses, and cloverleafs had not been invented. At each of these crossings stood a sign-post, topped by a white X, lettered in black with the words STOP, LOOK AND LISTEN. Sometimes people didn't stop ("I can make it!"); if they looked, they looked the other way; and no one knew afterwards to what they had been listening. There were accidents. Later, there were red wigwag signals and you could hear the signal bell at night as the train whistled for the crossing and roared on through. Accidents continued. Today, there are still accidents — at home, at play, on the high-ways, and at work — and for all the safety campaigns and safety belts, for all the statistics that document the human cost of accidental deaths and injuries, Americans act as though in truth they couldn't care less. It is high time that we recognize that accidents, like disease, are amenable to rational control meas-ures.

Accident prevention is an integral part of comprehensive per-sonal and environmental health services. Health leadership must increase its efforts to prevent accidental injuries, disabilities, and death. [F]

If the many groups and individuals who are already involved in accident prevention programs worked together, it would be possible to develop a program that included a wide variety of services: data collection and analysis on various kinds of acci-dents; continued review of possible legal controls; financial sup-port for demonstration projects; recruitment and training of personnel for the programs; public education about accident hazards and how to avoid them; special first-aid training for those who would deal with accidents at the source; improved community hospital facilities for emergency treatment of acci-dents; better transportation services for getting the injured to a place of treatment; extension of poison control centers as clearing houses for information to physicians and the public; enforcement of existing laws aimed at reducing hazards; and continuing re-search into all facets of the problem. The State Health Depart-ment should take the initiative in developing statewide accident prevention programs and eliciting the cooperation and support of other official and voluntary agencies. [F-1]

Research in all areas of accident prevention should be rapidly increased in amounts commensurate with the importance of the problem. Increased effort should be directed to those areas which have been generally neglected in the past, such as the home, the farm, and small industries, as well as to the major problems of making streets and highways safer for pedestrians, and automobiles safer for drivers and passengers. The United States Public Health Service should be given funds to establish a national accident prevention research, training service, and information facility analagous to the present Communicable Disease Center. [F-2]

Specialized reporting programs followed by investigation should be undertaken to furnish a body of statistics which will be of value in pointing out areas that demand the greatest concentration of research and action.

The present accident prevention efforts of voluntary agencies, associations, industry, and government should be encouraged and given increased financial support to assess and expand their programs in line with demonstrated needs and modern concepts [F-3], and there should be stricter enforcement of present laws and regulations designed to control or diminish accident hazards. [F-4] In its concern with accident prevention, the Commission has been aware that, of the many factors contributing to the accidental event, the human factor has been the one most neglected. To supplement current safety programs of industry, public transportation, and the National Safety Council, it is time for all other interested groups to accelerate work toward effective methods of accident prevention.

Progress in understanding the human factors in accidents is most likely to come from careful epidemiological studies. Epidemiology is the tool of the public health physician in much the way the X-ray machine is the tool of the diagnostician. Here lies one of the greatest opportunities for preventive medicine today. The epidemiological approach is as applicable to the study of accidents as it has proved to be in the study of disease.

Action involving three factors causes accidents: the person who is working, playing, or driving (the host); the automobile or other equipment in use (the agent); and environment. Physicians, because they have knowledge of the characteristics of people, can collaborate in analyzing causes of accidents and can also help to educate the person to prevent accidents — continuing meanwhile, as physicians always have, to treat the victims. Advance detection of accident-repeaters has yet to be perfected, but at least medical officers and industrial physicians can check on persons with a record of repeated accidents and determine through clinical methods how well adapted they are to their current activities. In terms of the potential "agent" in an accident, application of the principles of engineering can help to make men, their machines, and their interrelationships safer. Such engineering principles include the analysis of possible faults in the design of the equipment in relation to its use by man, and should be applied in conjunction with concern for the effect of physical change on the individual. Safe performance relates inexorably with changes in the level of light, of temperature and humidity, and with the presence of toxic agents such as carbon monoxide. In these situations there is generally well-defined knowledge of indoor levels at which man can operate safely and efficiently, and this knowledge, broadened to include outdoor levels, can be more widely disseminated and used.

There is also widespread knowledge of the effect that fatigue, worry, alcohol, or drugs have on a person's ability to perform safely. Although these effects are known, this knowledge is not fully utilized to reduce accidents. To control accidents in the same way they control preventable disease, physicians and health departments must cooperate with and have cooperation from all relevant enforcing agencies. Knowledge of the effect of alcohol on man's reflexes is of little use if the drunk-driving laws are not enforced, just as awareness of a man's fatigue horizon will not help him if the industry for which he works fails to provide rest periods at appropriate intervals and safety guards on its machines.

In a discussion of the total community health establishment, we should direct attention to the following figures which indicate how accidents increase the load on our health facilities: there are 52,000,000 people injured annually; 2,000,000 require hospitalization from injuries; 45,000,000 require some medical attention; 10,000,000 are bed-disabled; 65,000 hospital beds are required for treatment of accidents; and 88,000 hospital personnel are required for the treatment of accident victims.

In accident prevention, as in water and air pollution and other environmental problems discussed in this chapter, we must recognize that a properly managed environment is a positive force for health. Without that force, no amount of personal health services can keep people alive and well. With research, with scientific awareness and agreement, and with public support, there remains no substantive barrier to a clean and healthy environment for all of the people.

CHAPTER IV

The Consumer

There is a game called "Who Am I?" in which one person is "it." Everyone else asks him questions and the winner is the one whose question causes the subject to identify himself. The problems of identity, both for the consumers of health services and for those who provide them have to be considered seriously if communication and understanding are to be achieved as the foundation of a communitywide health service program. This game is for keeps.

Every individual shares certain common characteristics in relation to his attitudes toward health care: he is a human being, a person who reacts to symptoms of disease and the idea of disease itself with fears and anxieties that can cause other symptoms; he is a person who needs to learn how to lead a healthful life as well as how to recover from an illness; he needs advice and comfort and understanding; he needs to be loved. Knowledgeable men are saying this in many ways today as they search for methods to provide the people with the services they need, but the avenues of communication between health personnel and the people they treat are too often blocked by some aspects of the health system. Persons with little education and low income, sometimes hampered by barriers in language, are too often apprehensive, confused, or overwhelmed by scattered facilities and the impersonal and institutionalized services with which they are frequently confronted. They may be shunted from one clinic to another, one specialist to another, one laboratory to another; and their histories have to be repeated because the record fails to follow them. When this occurs, a man often rejects or is rejected by the only sources of aid available to him, and it takes a real crisis before he or his family looks again for help. Meanwhile, his problems have multiplied and are even more difficult to solve.

This lack of communication, and sometimes of trust, is by no means limited to the low-income groups and the non-English-speaking population. Large segments of the American public are confused in evaluating health and medical advice as "good," "adequate," or "quackery," and many — especially young people in their teens and twenties — are beginning to object to the use of fear techniques in the promotion of both medical products and preventive health habits, and to reject this sort of "advice." However, in spite of this confusion, most individuals will usually answer the "Who am I?" question to the best of their ability if they think that the questioner really cares. Only when those who provide health services know and understand the kinds of people they serve can they even begin to win the trust and cooperation of individual patients. We must concern ourselves with how the "providers" of health services are educated — not only substantively, but in their attitudes toward the consumer. Otherwise, in this computer culture that is springing up around us, the service will be a mere function — for the provider a service to be rendered by formula and with little feeling; for the consumer a service from a stranger. This is the core of the task facing the men and women who wish to build and administer a comprehensive health program providing continuity of care.

The computer has its own function, and it is a valuable one. To learn the collective and individual identities of America's new faces each year, the initial need is to expand both the collection of demographic data and its dissemination. Automation, specifically in terms of data collection and processing, provides us with the opportunity to discover many things we need to know about the population of any sector of this country. The door-to-door census takers can now be supplemented by the computers in providing a community profile. Investigators already know that by using electronic computer techniques they can quickly arrive at positive findings which, in many instances, could only be slowly approximated as recently as ten or fifteen years ago. Similar use should be made of data processing outside the laboratory, in regional centers, for example, where information on drugs, pathology, or treatment techniques can be obtained from laboratories, hospitals, universities, and public health departments, then stored and disseminated for use in local community facilities on demand. Health professionals need to develop the utilization of automated techniques, including the processing of statistics applicable to the analysis of human behavior and to conditions of environment and of disease, both general and specific. We already know more about the characteristics of the American people than has ever been known about a large population. This knowledge can serve as a starting point on which to base plans for the delivery of health services. What do we know? How do we interpret that knowledge? Who are we?

The American Population

We are the people of the United States of America who pledged our lives, our fortunes, and our sacred honor to, among many other things, promote the general welfare. "The general welfare" had fewer complexities in the eighteenth century than it has in the twentieth, but our present abundance of resources can be utilized to promote the welfare of a modern society made up as it is of a heterogeneous, growing, and shifting population. As more and more of our people move from the country to towns, cities, and metropolitan areas, these communities have a new set of problems to cope with in providing health services. Retiring farmers moving to small towns place a severe strain on the few services that exist there. Large numbers of people, young and old, moving to the larger cities pose other problems besides those caused by the numerical increase in population: frequently these groups have not had certain services available to them before and have little information about their eligibility for these services and less knowledge of how to acquire them. They compete for living space with other groups with extremely limited incomes, require an extensive array of services, and contribute little to the tax income to provide such services.

At the same time, many families moving to suburbia "for the children," take with them not only tax income from the city but top leadership in civic and political affairs. These leaders, who are policymakers for public and private agencies, soon lose touch with the needs and conditions of the population left in the city, and yet, to a substantial degree, they make the decisions about health services for these populations.

The consumers of health services range from the core city multicatastrophe family to the suburbanite executive — and most of them keep having children. As demographers and economists study the implications of population growth in relation to the gross national product, it appears that there is a consensus that, even though the size of the population will continue to increase, an economy as rich as ours can cope with the numerical increase for at least the next generation, if we will.

If we do not as yet face a crisis in the growth of the population, we do face a need for sharing, which can bring with it individual constraint, as we adapt to our environment. Our concern is with the acute problems of health, social welfare, and efficiency; and they are intrinsically related to significant developments within our population more important than mere numbers.

Between 1965 and 1970 the number of women aged 20 to 24 will increase by approximately 25 percent. This growth in the number of persons in the young, childbearing ages presages an increase in the number of births in the next five years. There are other factors tending in the opposite direction — indications that for all the childbearing age groups, the number of children expected per family may be beginning to decline. On balance, however, even if the size of the family becomes smaller, the number of babies born between 1965 and 1970 will undoubtedly be larger as a result of the growing numbers of potential parents.

Many of our problems stem from the heavy load of childbearing carried by those segments of the population who have the lowest social and economic resources — largely the minority groups. These are not the people who have contributed the largest numbers to the postwar rise in births. The largest numerical increase came from the middle class of the population. But the gross measurements by either numbers or percentages are less important than the fact that a poverty-stricken and poorly educated sector of the population, representing some 30,000,000 people, is reproducing at rates almost comparable with those of parts of Asia, at a time when repeated investigations show that most of them have more children than they want. These are the people who need the most and are least able to provide their children the health, education, housing, income, and family stability that must serve as the background for effective participation in modern American life. Victims of this situation are in many instances Negroes, members of Spanish-speaking groups, or poorly educated newcomers to cities who grew up in rural poverty. There is no evidence that their problems are intrinsically caused by their race or their language. Nineteenth-century immigrants from Ireland, Italy, and Poland had the same problems when they were economic and social minorities because this country allowed them to subsist in intolerable living conditions. We are now faced with the social disorganization resulting from large pockets of poverty, and we are beginning to realize that we must invest heavily in methods to provide for better health and education.

Agreement has not been reached in terms of provision of the means to control population growth, but attitudes are changing and today one of the major dialogues occurring in the health field is the debate on population or birth control. (Who am I? I am a young American who likes children. I want some of my own. I want them to have a good home and education. But I think how many I have and when I have them is a matter of personal freedom. Everybody else I know feels the same way, but nobody tells me what I need to know. I want to have babies and I want to know how to bring them up right. That's who I am.)

Along with the past century's growing scientific knowledge about human reproduction and emphasis on human freedom and human responsibility has come increasing recognition that family planning is an essential component of individual and family health and contributes to a healthy community.

Family planning should be an integral part of community health services. Private and public health agencies must accept responsibility for the provision of family planning services and for the support of scientific research on human fertility. Family planning is essential to individual and family health and contributes to a healthy community. All individuals have the right to have convenient access to information about the different methods available and to practice those methods acceptable to them for the benefit of their offspring, their family life, and their community. [G]

The issues of family planning are beginning to rise to the top in public debate in this country. This in itself is healthy, and the Commission believes that public and private programs concerned with population control should be integral parts of the health program. Because of the impact of population changes on health, scientific research on human fertility and on the related factors influencing population changes should be immediately intensified. [G-1] Further, instruction in family planning should be a routine health service carried out in appropriate facilities by qualified personnel. [G-2]

The Commission has not included intensive work on family planning in its studies, since many other groups are currently doing so. It agrees, however, that the central goal is to improve the practices of family planning, and concurs with the following suggestions put forward by the Population Council: (1) Offer family planning information to every obstetrical patient and give help to any patient requesting it at the time of the postpartum check, with due respect for religious beliefs. (2) Make family planning a part of the health services offered by each hospital to its outpatients. (3) Make family planning advice and services an integral part of the various plans for medical care. (4) Instruct and allow every social worker employed by either public or private agencies to deal with the problems of family planning in the same way that other family problems are discussed and solved.

Such rather simple innovations would go far toward solving the problem of unwanted children and family disorganization in the most depressed sectors of the population, and would make acceptable and available information and practices which, although widely utilized in middle- and high-income groups, are currently circumscribed by legal and medical taboos.

Population Density

In addition to family planning, individuals and groups concerned with environmental stress and with ugliness and beauty are studying not so much the numbers of people in the nation but the density in which they congregate and live.

Planning for a healthy environment is an essential consideration in urban design. Immediate steps must be taken by those responsible for the control of land use, transportation, economic development, and related physical and social planning to coordinate their activities to: provide for the most effective use of space for our rapidly growing urban population; avoid ill effects that may be associated with high population densities; reduce hazards to physical and emotional health from overcrowding where it exists; and contribute to an aesthetically and emotionally satisfying environment conducive to positive health. [H]

Nearly three-fourths of our population will be urban dwellers during the last quarter of this century. Some sections of the nation, embracing several states, will soon be broad belts of high population density. The urban center is fast becoming the metropolitan area, and several metropolitan areas are merging into the megalopolis. The effects of so many people living so close together need attention now in order to prevent those effects that contribute to ill health and make good use of those that enhance life.

Studies of the effects of crowding indicate that the amount of living room, or space, available is a highly important factor both in causing and reducing stress. Current studies show that the need for privacy may prove to be just as basic as the need for food, sex, and approval. We are learning more about the effects of slum living on the people who live there as we go about modern urban renewal activities. In view of the close association of ill health and poverty, the Commission recommends that immediate steps be taken to make the full range of health services of the community (with emphasis on programs of prevention and rehabilitation) available and acceptable for those who live in areas which combine high population density, chronic poverty, and deprivation. [H-1]

We are also learning more about isolation and poverty as we progress in the economic and social programs initiated by legislation that activated the poverty program and the program for Appalachian development. Our knowledge is still imprecise and further research is needed both in the behavioral sciences and in the relationships between physical environment and health. However, if the findings of certain widely known studies of animals other than man are applicable to human populations, it is reasonable to assume that the effects of crowding are usually detrimental and may in some situations affect the behavior of an entire group, causing the death rate to rise and the birth rate to fall. Although man has yet to discover the degree to which such crowding affects him, we have had enough experience in prisons, concentration camps, and areas which, although not enclosed by fences, limited the freedom of the inhabitants through poverty, to realize that the crowding of increased urbanization is a potential hazard to both physical and emotional health. The Department of Housing and Urban Development and the United States Department of Health, Education, and Welfare should take primary responsibility in cooperation with other appropriate federal agencies and voluntary and professional organizations in developing criteria to measure the effect of population mobility, density, and urban conditions on the physical, emotional, and social health of people; and in promoting research and experimentation in urban design, land use, and population distribution as these relate to health. [H-2]

Additionally, more and more architects, landscape designers, and artists are assembling data to substantiate their belief that an aesthetically happy man is often a healthy man. These men want to plan and design our environments so that man can walk in beauty as he goes about his daily work. This is certainly no new idea; industries have proved the correlation between pleasant surroundings and productivity; hospitals have demonstrated the relation between pleasant surroundings and recovery; architects have designed buildings which house hundreds of people in filing cabinet adjacency, yet still provide the illusion of space and the great outdoors. The nation's current quest in this area is mainly one of adapting its creativity to individual and community economics.

But it is not a simple thing to adapt creativity and economics, for one man's economic interests can change the physical face of an entire community. Highway engineers, men who construct entire community tracts as self-sufficient communities, and others have at times ignored the common good for personal gain. This "environment-be-damned" attitude seems to be changing, however, as more and more industrialists and community builders realize that it is to their own economic interests to accept their share of the responsibility to maintain a healthy environment and a beautiful one. Public health authorities must actively enforce statutes and standards designed for public safety and must control activities whose attendant noise, dust, and land-eroding effects are against the public interest.

There is an urgent need for the development of model legislation that would require all programs related to physical city planning (for example, land use, urban design and renewal, highway construction, public housing) to provide for the healthful distribution of population; protection from hazardous, noisy, and unaesthetic environments; availability and accessibility of comprehensive health and welfare services; and space for recreational and cultural activities. [H-3]

Too often in the past, even though the laws were on the books, the public health officer either lacked initiative or did not receive the support of his community as he tried to enforce the controls available to him. Today's health crises make it imperative that communities give their health officers effective support, and that their health officers are trained to recognize the widening perimeters of their job.

Individual Responsibility for Health

In stating that the community — of whatever size and sufficiency — has a responsibility to provide accessible health services of high quality, the Commission in no way implies that the responsibility stops here. Every person, to the extent of his knowledge, must assume responsibility for his continuing good health. The key words here, however, are "to the extent of his knowledge." If in our American society, we assume that the people have a right to know, where can they go for education about health?

Who will be the teacher, who the student, and in what classrooms will they meet? Effective health education must be available to the individual of all ages, the family, and the entire community. Health education must begin and must continue to reach people where they are — at their current level of awareness of personal and community health matters. Such education, to be effective, must teach basic health knowledge, attitudes, and practices, and the teaching must cause the student to act — either to do something because it will promote his health or to refrain from doing something that will be hazardous to him or to those around him.

Education for health is a fundamental aspect of community health services and is basic to every health program. It should stimulate each individual to assume responsibility for maintaining personal health through life and to participate in community health activities. The community has a responsibility for developing an organized and continuing educational program concerning health resources for its residents. Each individual has a personal responsibility for making full use of available resources. [I]

Health education can and should be provided in varying degree by many kinds of people. The major problem has been brought about by the fact that the people who teach about health are not quite sure where their job begins and where it ends. The health educator can provide special services to many sectors of the community. The physician can explain the nature of illness and treatment to his patients and he can also explain preventive measures. The housewife can teach her family and recommend a course of action to her neighbor. The teacher can teach the rules of personal and public health to students. Voluntary health agencies can further develop public education programs relating to the agency's field of interest. Special interest groups within a community can identify their specific objectives in health education and coordinate their work with the work of others.

None of these concepts is new. What is new is that communities are now becoming aware of the fact that knowledge about health, like knowledge in any other field, must be taught so as to motivate the person receiving the information to relate it to himself and to his own life.

The objectives for health education, then, are to interest each individual in his own health and the means to improve it; to teach him where health services are available; to motivate him to use them; and to enable him to discriminate between scientific health care and quackery.

All settings for health education are major — at home, at

school, at work, and within the community and its health facilities.

At home. Health education for each member of the family begins at home and is practiced there. Unfortunately much of the practice is less than good, but the fact remains the families still provide a great deal of health care for their members, and that care, or lack of it, is based on information and attitudes coming into the home through all manner of communication. These include what Johnny said the teacher told him at school; what somebody read in a newspaper, heard on the radio, or saw on TV; what another member of the family, or a friend, saw in an advertisement; what Mrs. Smith said yesterday at the supermarket; and, most important, the behavior of parents and other adults who come into the home. They should also include information provided by the community's official, voluntary, and professional health organizations, as well as consumer and civic groups concerned with health and education.

Health education must come closer to the people. This will occur as more personal health services become more readily available, and as the people who provide the services secure the confidence of the population by further adapting their services to the people's needs. This nation is currently concerned with the improvement of all kinds of education for all kinds of people. It is imperative that, while bringing the three "R's" to more people, education about the big "H" — health — be included in our new plans for learning.

At school. No one is really to be blamed that health education has become fragmented and superficial in most communities. Education for health has been everybody's business and no one's clear responsibility. In many school curriculums, for example, teachers have been required to work something called "health education" into a few hours of the physical education period each year. Many employers have assumed that, as long as an employee was at work, he was healthy. For too many people, the image of "public health" was projected mainly by such things as signs in subways which informed them that "spitting is unhealthy and breeds disease."

The teacher of health, like the teacher of any other subject, must know something about the people he teaches, as well as the subject to be taught. ("Who am I? I'm a kid in school. They tell me something about physical fitness, but mostly its 50-mile hikes or training for the team. When they talk about cigarette smoking, drinking, or marijuana, or taking dope or glue-sniffing, I don't think most of them know the straight stuff; they act as though they teach about drinking because they have to. And the way they teach sex education, it should never happen to you! They have good classes in drivers' education and shop; if you want to, you can learn history and English and math from teachers. But, if you really want to know anything about 'health,' you learn it from the other kids.")

Health education must become a fundamental part of the basic, balanced curriculum; it can be effectively taught in school, and no other public agency today offers health instruction to children of school age. State Departments of Education and local school boards should assume greater responsibility for the development of health curriculums. In so doing, the schools should look to health departments and voluntary health agencies for assistance in providing continuity and resources. [I-1] Such combinations of community health resources and professional experience can supplement the school's program and help provide a meaningful health learning experience for students and teachers.

At work. Health education, like other aspects of health, is a lifetime thing. The time and place of employment present significant occasions for health promotion. Among these are industrial safety and accident prevention programs, pre-employment and periodic health examinations, health insurance interpretation and utilization, screening tests for early detection and immunization programs — each of which should encompass continuing educational elements.

Health departments and voluntary health agencies should make available resources for health education programs in business and industry. These resources should be utilized to supplement in-plant health information and counseling efforts. [I-2]

In the community. Every health care agency and facility has as many opportunities to provide health education as there are patients. When a person is in a physician's office, a dentist's office, a clinic, or an emergency room, he may be far more "teachable" than at other times when he feels fine and has his mind on other things. Health personnel, traditionally overworked and hurried, must be given the opportunity to include positive health education for prevention of disease in their discussion with the patient.

Obviously there is need for better health services information and referral mechanisms. Equally obvious is the need for co-ordinating health education services not merely to avoid over-lapping but to bridge gaps and serve emerging needs and population groups. Many of the more important gaps can be bridged by the active involvement of people — those served as well as those serving and helping to serve. Major obstacles to constructive use of health resources have been cultural barriers, not only between middle-class-oriented professional staff and those seeking service, but between the traditional concepts of health services for the "indigent" and those for the more affluent sectors of the community.

Person-to-person contact as a basic implement in effective communication does not, however, reduce the importance of wider application of other means of communication and educa-tion. Manifest abuses in the use of the mass media do not obviate the fact that the press, radio, television, and advertising — the latter notably through the Advertising Council — have con-tributed significantly to constructive health education. The chal-lenge to the health community is to understand these channels and to offer opportunities for collaboration between industry and control agencies in the public interest. This goes beyond preventing the basically fraudulent, untrue, or misleading com-mercials that have not been banished from the airways or printed page because of a saving phrase or qualification easily ignored by its hearers or readers. It also means spotting the innuendo and the half-truth which self-policing has failed to avoid. The occasional public service program or feature dedicated to a scrupulously honest presentation of a health issue is a step in the right direction. Health educators can do much to assure the constructive use of public communications media to improve health.

In short, if individuals are to be expected to accept their

responsibilities for health for themselves, their families, and their communities, the health and education agencies of the community must reach out to them and establish the kind of understanding that fosters individual action.

Innovation and Research

To realize these goals will require imaginative new programs, additional experimentation and innovation, and use of newer techniques and methods arising in other fields of education and technology. Aggressive, pragmatic health education programs must be created and fitted to special needs. More applied research in educational techniques and methods must be undertaken to supplement and draw from physical and social science research findings, particularly those which apply to health attitudes, motivation, and behavior. [I-3]

Perhaps the most frustrating of all the frustrations experienced by those concerned with health education is the behavioral gap between what people know is good for their health and what they actually do. Between the child's "Gee, Mom, I know I should'a brushed my teeth, but the guys were waiting for me!" and his father's deliberate enjoyment of a second piece of pie after too much dinner, the behavioral distance is nil. We understand too little but we apply less than we know. The opportunities for constructive research and application are vast. Their development should parallel our efforts in medical and administrative research.

In the past, "health education" has been divided between two teams — the public health educators and the school health educators. Granted there is need for individuals whose specialty may be one or the other, education for health is too basic to comprehensive health services to allow for outmoded divisions of territory among its practitioners. All health education personnel should be given courses covering the needs of the rapidly expanding health field, including administration, community organization, and action-planning. [I-4] Schools of public health should maintain a department or unit specializing in relevant areas of education and communication. Schools of public health and schools of education should cooperate in training health educators. [I-5]

Health "Quackery"

The principle that guides the medical profession was stated in less than 50 words. "A Physician," said Hippocrates, "should be an upright man, instructed in the art of healing — modest, sober, patient, prompt to do his whole duty without anxiety; pious without going so far as superstition, conducting himself with propriety in his profession and in all the actions of his life."

The health quack looks to no such guideposts; instead, since early times, he has been preying on the undiscerning, the uninformed, the desperate, the unsuspecting of all ages. To prevent such encroachments, concerted action must be taken through law enforcement, legislation, and education to limit the practice of medicine to those who are scientifically educated and licensed. Quality health care should be the goal for Americans. The public should be advised by all possible means and methods that this can be obtained only from scientifically trained practitioners. Health educators, professional organizations, and official and voluntary health agencies must intensify their efforts to inform the public of the hazards to the health and wealth of this nation posed by quack and cult practitioners. [B-4]

Joined by the cultists, the health quacks are in business today, bilking people of millions of dollars a year. Estimates of the costs of medical quackery in dollars are at best calculated guesses but they run as high as a billion dollars a year. In terms of lives, one authority in health education has stated that medical quackery each year costs more lives than all the crimes in the United States. It is this cost of life and impaired health to which the people of the United States must be alerted. For one insidious side effect of quackery in all its sordid forms is the delay in obtaining effective medical care — a delay that can cost life itself. The cultists, who turn their backs on scientific medicine, must accept equal responsibility with the quacks for producing these health hazards.

The licensure of the health professions and supportive occupations has expanded over the years as the numbers and kinds of training programs and the scope of their services have changed. Individual state legislatures have responded differently as pressures for licensure and recognition have differed. The role of accreditation of the educational requirements for the various health programs has varied widely. It is apparent that the certification of the educational requirement for degrees or certificates by established accrediting bodies should be expanded.

The rapid development of the health services and the expansion of the health sciences will create new service opportunities and professions for which licensure and accreditation will be required, and we are in need of a model code, that states could adopt, that would provide for uniform licensure of the health professions. Such a code should be developed without delay by a national citizens commission. [B-4]

Consumer Health Protection

Probably nothing in the health field has become more complicated than consumer health protection — protection from infection and provision of a safe and uncontaminated food and drug supply. Occasionally public concern reaches a climax, when a drug such as thalidomide causes the malformation of thousands of babies, or the improper processing of eggs results in widespread salmonella infection. But usually the American public rests in happy confidence that somehow, between industry, voluntary agencies, and government, safe standards will be enforced and all will be well. The fact is that we have by no means achieved a procedure that guarantees that all food, drugs, and therapeutic devices are safe. Industry, appropriate voluntary agencies, and government must increase cooperation in developing the scientific and technical resources that are needed to improve controls of the food and drug supply and to protect both the public and industry itself by keeping injurious products off the market.

Regulations to provide pure food and nutritious food begin long before the food goes into the package. We do not know all the effects on humans of the chemicals which are now used routinely as part of food production and protection. Nor do we know the long-range effect of the many other physical and chemical agents — solvents, plastics, herbacides, and isotopes, for example. Research by government and industry must be substantially increased to determine the immediate and long-range cumulative effects of radiological techniques and of physical, biological, and chemical products on man, to plan for and conduct education and enforcement programs, and to keep pace with the new technology. [E-9]

Without waiting for the results of that research, however, it is imperative that special measures be taken to teach the consumer to avoid the misuse of physical, biological, and chemical products now available for use in the home, on the farm, and in industry. Such products as solvents, pesticides, plastics, and devices involving the use of microwaves, should be labeled as to correct storage and use; they should be systematically tested; and, if necessary, their distribution should be continuously monitored. [E-10]

Industry, governments, voluntary agencies, educational institutions, and communications media must join in the development of continuous and effective education programs designed to inform the public of the danger of pollutant activities and the steps to be taken to avoid them. We must develop easily recognizable signals for alerting the public to the level of air and water pollutants (like the smog-level signals now in use in Los Angeles, or the fire-danger levels used by national parks) and publish and dramatize through all media how to respond to these warning signals. [E-11]

Just as the drug industry is required by the Food and Drug Administration to test the safety of its own products, the federal government should require manufacturers of pesticides and other economic chemicals to assume the burden of proof that their products are not harmful to human life if properly used. [E-12] Industry is becoming more receptive to this sort of self-policing, since the errors or carelessness of one producer can often damage the entire industry — as has been demonstrated by the cranberry and canned tuna scares.

All measures designed for the protection of the total population cannot be secured by any one consumer; every man must rely on governmental authority to provide certain controls. At present, there are far too many overlapping agencies at every level of government and within the private sector of the community, each with authority and responsibility. Communities, in the best interests of the residents who pay for and expect protection, must arrive at new approaches to weld the many agencies concerned with protection into a more effective and responsible entity.

The Cost to the Consumer

Not so long ago, one of the standard jokes in the folklore of this country was about paying the doctor's bill last. The long-suffering medical profession has adopted modern payment procedures which, in most instances, force the consumer of personal health services to pay up as promptly as he pays the installment on his car or the grocery bill; but, since the cost of all health services cannot be individually budgeted, the consumer needs help in paying for his health. Until it happens to them personally, most people are not aware of the fact that in some state hospitals patients are still required to sign a lien on any real property in which they may have an equity before they are given even emergency treatment. The Medicare legislation removes this fear for those it covers, but others in need of lengthy treatment in state hospitals may postpone that treatment because they know that a lien will be placed on their home in the amount of the total cost of their treatment. Voluntary health agencies and citizens' groups throughout the country are working to change such restrictive legislation, claiming that it penalizes the lower middle income group in the population. Nowhere does the "middle-class squeeze" show up more dramatically than in the case of catastrophic or chronic illness. The indigent, if they demand it, can receive treatment for which the salaried worker could not possibly pay. One answer, of course, is health insurance, Blue Cross, and other prepayment plans. Such plans are an effective method for financing a major part of personal health service, even though many of them are still inadequate in the scope of services covered.

The nation has yet to feel the impact of Medicare. Obviously, more health services will now be financed for persons over 65 years of age, but what of the person aged 64, or 23? The young and middle-aged consumers of health services are the groups which pay the largest share of the nation's taxes. If population projections are correct, these are the groups who will be paying for the health care of more babies and of more nonproductive elderly people in the next five to ten years. It is imperative, therefore, that methods of financing health services, from the point of view of the consumer, as well as from that of those who provide the services, must be immediately given more intensive attention by legislators, tax experts, and private prepayment plans. Prepayment and insurance plans must develop mechanisms for financing the health services included in a comprehensive care program. Today's modern consumer must be able to purchase protection to meet at least a proportion of the cost of preventive services, dentistry, rehabilitation, home care, care at the physician's office and the outpatient clinic, nursing home and extended care, as well as care provided in a hospital.

This generation has witnessed a phenomenal expansion in a variety of mechanisms developed to assist the consumer in meeting the costs of medical care. From the beginning, this expansion has been most prominent among employed groups where protection can be most readily provided through the employment relationship and where the tax structure lends encouragement to it. Some provision for health protection has now become the most widely accepted fringe benefit both in collective bargaining and in programs initiated by employers.

More than 1800 organizations sell health insurance to the American public. Included are 900 commercial stock or mutual insurance companies selling individual and group insurance; 150 Blue Cross and Blue Shield plans, affiliated in varying degrees with hospital associations and medical societies respectively; and nearly 800 so-called independent plans, including community- and consumer-sponsored plans, and the health insurance programs of union welfare funds, employers, employee organizations, and physicians. Participation in the integrated program of health service should continue to be financed from a variety of sources, including out-of-pocket payments, insurance and prepayment plans, and public funds. [B-10]

This wide variety of arrangements reflects several quite different approaches to the problem of health care and personal health financing, each with its own advantages and disadvantages which must be understood and evaluated both in terms of the specific needs each is designed to meet and in terms of the broad public interest in their development.

The early plans were based primarily on the concept of sickness and its attendant costs being an insurable risk which could be met by spreading such risk through insurance plans or policies that provided the insured with cash to pay medical bills at the time of illness. This basic concept remains in indemnity health insurance, though there has been developed a wide variety of plans within the category. Usually, like any other insurance, the entire cost of the illness is not recoverable; thus, the insured must carry part of the risk.

This approach has a number of advantages. It is completely portable, its benefits, being in cash, provide the insured varying degrees of protection wherever he may be when he needs it. It has self-policing features, discouraging overutilization by the insured, since he must carry part of the cost out-of-pocket. Where the cost of the plan is borne in whole or in part by an employer, the employer has a motive to help prevent overutilization, since his premium rates are related to utilization rates. These plans give the insured complete freedom of choice of physician or health institution providing service. Since the benefits are in stated dollar amounts, the costs of the programs are predictable and controllable.

The shortcomings of these programs are chiefly: though overutilization is discouraged on the part of the insured, it may actually be encouraged on the part of the providers of services; while providing freedom of choice, they give the insured consumer no guidance or help in the area of greatest consumer confusion and in an area that has no accepted consumer standards; and, through the coinsurance principle, early diagnosis, preventive health care, and even treatment services may be discouraged.

Also among the early protection methods were the service plans, of which Blue Cross is typical. Here the benefit is not in cash to pay bills, but the service itself which is paid for by the plan. These have the advantage of portability, since the nation is now blanketed with plans, practically all of which have reciprocal arrangements. The plans have some influence on cost as they are in a position to bargain to a certain extent with the providers of service. In recent years more of these plans have joined with the providers of service in controlling overutilization, and the potential for further efforts of this kind exists within their framework. Service and indemnity plans are expanding their benefits. Both have the disadvantage inherent in the shared cost for diagnosis and treatment of disease. Both indemnity and benefit plans are available through nonprofit organizations, such as Blue Cross, and in a wide variety of combinations through commercial insurance carriers.

An outgrowth of the basic insurance approach, but differing in a number of important respects, are the "direct service" group practice prepayment plans, which have their own medical staff and facilities and which provide services "directly" to their enrolled members. The insurance concept is adhered to in these plans only to the extent that the costs are spread among its members, and over a period of time. The benefits, however, are not confined to a period of illness. More basic than the insurance concept is that of budgeting through regular payments to cover the entire costs of medical care, including prevention, cure, and rehabilitation. The plan profits, too, since such comprehensive care tends to reduce the incidence of the more expensive types of medical service, such as surgery and hospitalization.

The disadvantages are chiefly that such plans are limited geographically, and reciprocal arrangements among them have not been fully worked out; protection, therefore, is far from being completely portable. The member does not have complete freedom of choice, since the physicians available to him are limited to those affiliated with the plan. Many feel, however, that this is more than compensated for by the fact that the physician who serves the individual is selected by other physicians, who are far more likely to be knowledgeable about his qualifications.

Where the goal is complete coverage, with comprehensive health care, the prepayment plans, coupled with a group practice program, may have distinct advantages. These prepaid, group practice plans are not, however, available to all consumers. Some states have restrictive legislation which either forbids or impedes their development. The Commission believes that these legal restrictions should be removed, and that full experimentation with such plans should be encouraged. [B-11]

The potentials for comprehensive coverage among the indemnity and direct service plans have not been exhausted by any means. With all the efforts among all the various types of nongovernmental plans which now provide some protection to more than 70 percent of the population, less than one-third of personal health expenditures are now being met by such plans.

Participation in the various types of plans designed to meet the variety of individual and varying group needs should be extended. Some may continue to prefer out-of-pocket payment at the time of illness. For most of the population, however, health insurance should be developed or extended to provide protection — whether they are employed, self-employed, or unemployed — for them and for their dependents. All interested parties should pursue this extension of coverage by all possible methods, including the appropriate use of public monies. Health insurance should cover out-of-hospital care as well as in-hospital care, and it must cover the full range of services: preventive, diagnostic, therapeutic, and rehabilitative for both mental and physical illness. [B-10]

The entire consideration of expansion of prepayment plans, however, continues in a period of sudden change whose effects cannot as yet be measured. Major factors on which rates are based include: benefits, utilization, controls, provider costs, and the impact of government programs covering selected segments of the population. The Commission believes that rigorous examination of these factors should be undertaken by the plans before rate changes are proposed and by rate-setting authorities reviewing proposals. [B-12]

Blue Cross plans, having been chartered by special enactments of the state legislatures, present particular public policy issues. Blue Cross began as a hospital-sponsored and hospital-operated system. Today's needs indicate, however, that an agency which includes hospitals, subscribers, and the general public and assigns them equal representation in setting the plan's policy would meet the current need to give subscribers a larger say. At the same time, consumer representation on the policy-making board would provide a means to mediate differences between the hospital and the subscribers in the public interest. Such a balanced policy-making group would help assure prepaid insurance policies that are responsive to the needs of the whole community. A 1964 survey of the composition of the boards of trustees of Blue

Cross plans showed that 41 percent were public representatives with no hospital connection, 17 percent were also on the board of trustees of a hospital, 26 percent were hospital administrators, and 16 percent were physicians. These data reflect a continuing trend toward increased public representation which has been speeded by state legislation.

The establishment of regional health communities may be hindered unless Blue Cross plans are consolidated. Certain area differentials may reflect desirable local efforts and features, but, in the main, it is difficult for a plan covering a community of fewer than 500,000 people to achieve the quality of management necessary for effective operation, and there should be further study of the potential value of consolidation.

The complexity of modern medical care makes any artificial compartmentalization of insurances an impediment to unified, effective, and economical patient care. Nonprofit health insurance plans should have the opportunity to offer a broad range of services under their own auspices and within their own facilities if they so desire.

It is important to the interest of the community as a whole, as well as to the individual, that the cost of care for those who properly need and use larger amounts of care should be shared by all subscribers. Within the voluntary sector in the past this has been accomplished largely through community rating in the direct service and prepayment plans. Recently, there has been a significant movement toward experience rating where there is less sharing of protection for the high user. In pursuit of an economic objective, social objectives have been compromised. Recognizing this, plans have developed intermediate forms of class rating through which there are broad groupings of subscribers and provision is made for subsidization of the disadvantaged. To provide protection for the high-risk subscriber, the Commission favors either community rating or a type of class rating that accomplishes the same purpose. [B-12]

At the present time, one-half of all health and medical expenditures is met by consumers out-of-pocket and one-half is met through health insurance, tax funds, and philanthropy. This ratio will change, of course, as the result of the 1965 amendments to the Social Security Act and the implementation of the "heart,

cancer, and stroke" legislation. The ratio should also change
to benefit the consumer of health services and the provider of
those services, as prepayment and other health insurance programs are expanded to include more out-of-hospital treatment
situations, in both physical and mental illness. The protection
provided the individual by health insurance is obvious, but
another result of expanding insurance programs will be the
ability to expand private payment for health care and reduce the
amount of tax funds spent for personal health care. Certainly
for the population under age 65, expansion of voluntary health
insurance must continue.

Today's consumer knows that some things are missing from a
complete program of health services, and in many communities
consumers are taking a more active part with the professionals
to plan health programs that will identify and supply the missing
links.

CHAPTER V

Health Manpower

Three million men and women, comprising 4 percent of the total labor force in the United States, were employed in health services in 1964 — a sizable community of interest in itself. Considering that the delivery of health services constitutes one of the nation's largest enterprises, and that this enterprise has developed without conscious planning, it is not surprising that the separate services within the community are diverse and often have conflicting interests.

The Commission is concerned with the need to build a community of interest from this diversity. The concept of comprehensive health services it recommends provides for a new framework into which health services — personal and environmental — would fit, not in patchwork fashion, but through the achievement of an interdependent functioning entity within and among communities. In translating this concept into reality, health personnel will play a highly significant, in fact determining, role.

Through research men learn new things. If this knowledge results in better service to human beings, man, being human, wants access to such services in his search for improved quality of living. It is this chain reaction to which the people who provide health services address themselves as we look toward the twenty-first century.

The lapsed time between the day when Koch proved that many diseases could be traced to microorganisms and the day when man's ability to split the atom resulted in the creation of the field of nuclear medicine is an extremely brief historical period. Within it, medical research has brought about effective control, and even the eradication, of many diseases. Knowledge of antisepsis and asepsis, of anesthesia, of the X ray, of blood transfusions is joined with the ability to use cobalt therapy, radioactive isotopes, computers, and psychoactive drugs within an almost overwhelming variety of techniques and settings to serve man. The very size of this horn of plenty is a fundamental cause of the problems now evident.

Hand in hand with medical research and its ability to control diseases which have plagued mankind over centuries is the changing nature of man's environment and the broadening scientific base for the control of such hazards. The past several decades have seen greater concentrations of human beings in metropolitan areas, increasing radiological hazards to health, contamination of air and water through chemical pollutants, and increased hazards through the tremendous numbers of automobiles as well as changes in methods of farming and in the way men earn a living, either at the machine or on the farm.

Comprehensive community planning for all health services — personal and environmental — requires that these problems become the concern of the doctor, lawyer, and merchant chief, but the health professions must accept the greatest share of responsibility to improve health services, maintain quality care, and meet the needs of the entire community. The reports of the Commission's task forces have called attention to the need for altered relationships between health professionals and the allied and technical manpower who supply health services. Social changes are occurring within the health team itself. The explosion of medical and scientific knowledge in the past two or three decades has been so fast that it has precipitated a high degree of specialization, not only in medicine, but in the allied health professions as well. As knowledge increases, further specialization is inevitable. Among the primary issues is that of not losing sight of the total patient — or, for that matter, the entire community. The paramount need is for physicians and other members of the personal health care team to be especially trained to deal with the whole patient, in his social and environmental context. It is important that they understand the particular skills and contributions of each of the allied health professions and supporting personnel and know how to collaborate constructively with them. Their combined efforts must be integrated around the patient to meet his social and emotional as well as physical needs. This is also applicable to the health administrator, the engineer, or the scientist. It is essential, whether the health team be for the provision of personal health or environmental health services, to clarify the duties of each member, to determine the skills required of each, to insure appropriate training, and not to assign duties below the level of such training and competence.

The People Problem

The effective utilization of available health personnel will reduce the current manpower shortage, and continuous evaluation of use of manpower, accompanied by necessary changes and retraining, will provide additional manpower for existing and new health services. However, to provide comprehensive community health services in the next decade will require an unprecedented effort to recruit, educate, and train additional manpower for the health team. Such an effort should be intensive, planned, and continuous and should emphasize teamwork among all levels of health manpower. [J]

Every community must have available the skills and techniques of many kinds of health personnel. These needs are increasing in terms of numbers of people as well as kinds of skills required. The wide range of manpower for environmental and personal health service includes not only engineers and physicians, but many varieties of laboratory technicians, dentists, nurses, pharmacists, physical, occupational, and speech therapists, homemakers, health aides, social workers, psychological and vocational counselors, and nutritionists.

This nation has a chronic health problem: the chronic shortage of health personnel in all categories. The size of the shortage can only be estimated because the problem is compounded by uneven distribution and less than maximum utilization. The subtleties of the problem undoubtedly transcend the classic interactions of supply and demand, but we must face the fact that comprehensive information for the nation as a whole on the supply, distribution, and use of manpower simply is not available. As the initial step toward sound planning for recruitment, education, and use, we must find out more than we now know about health manpower. The Public Health Service should assume responsibility for collecting and reporting health manpower data on a nationwide basis, using standardized classifications, in cooperation with associations representing health occupations, educational institutions, and voluntary health agencies. [J-1]

We can be fairly sure of some general figures. For example, the number of physicians has doubled in the United States since 1900, the number of dentists has tripled, and the number of professional or college-trained health personnel of all kinds has increased six times, while the total population was increasing by two and a half. The rate of increase in the number of persons entering health activities in the future will depend on how attractive we make the training and the career to today's grammar and high school students as they prepare for further training — collegiate or technical — in any one of the hundreds of pursuits open to them. We must also make the best use of the talent we already have; additional public and private funds must be devoted to experiments and demonstrations to increase the productivity of all types of health personnel and improve the range and quality of service. [J-2]

In addition, each community must be able to enter the recruitment competition with the knowledge that financial reimbursement for all kinds of health personnel will be competitive with that received by people performing comparable jobs in the community. Wages for salaried professional, semiprofessional, and hourly-paid workers in the health field have improved substantially during the past decade, but are still generally below those paid for comparable skill and training elsewhere in the community. This gap must be closed if the best qualified personnel is to be recruited and retained. Hospitals and other health institutions, for example, are finding that, in a period of nearly full employment, manpower needs cannot be met by reliance on low-paid personnel available to them because of traditional exemption from wage and hour laws. Wage and hour laws and other protective legislation should be amended to include health personnel wherever their place of employment. [J-3]

Freedom of choice is a national precept, and the exercise of that choice is a large factor in determining the number of people who will decide to enter a health profession. Adequate salaries, favorable working conditions, and the opportunity for reward-ing, creative work are equally important in the fierce and demanding competition for recruits for the health field.

Statistics are illustrative, rather than complete, and indicate only one measure of the magnitude of the problem. At the end of 1965 the United States had 292,000 M.D.'s and 13,000 D.O.'s, for a total of 305,000 physicians, or 153 physicians for every 100,000 persons. To maintain this ratio, we will need about 352,000 physicians by 1975, assuming a population of 230,-000,000 at that time. While this figure may be met or exceeded if the present rate of influx of foreign medical graduates con-tinues, it could not be met by the projected growth in graduates of our own medical schools. The current figure of 7,800 graduates is expected to approach 10,000 by 1974, but would have to be much greater if our need for physicians were to be met entirely by American school graduates. Assumption of responsibility to train physicians for service in other countries would require still greater increases.

The ratio of active dentists for every 100,000 civilians declined from 49.9 in 1950 to 44.9 in 1963. In 1962, 550,000 professional nurses were practicing, but 117,000 of them were working only part-time. This supply must be considered in relation to the esti-mate prepared for the Surgeon General in 1963, that the nation would need 850,000 practicing professional nurses by 1975. This would require the graduating of 100,000 nurses annually by 1969; 1965's 33,200 graduates of schools of nursing were expected to provide a net addition of only 10,000 nurses, since 23,000 were expected to leave the profession.

The national supply of physical therapists is 10,000 and the estimated need is for 15,000. There are 7,500 qualified occupa-tional therapists available, but only approximately half of them are active in the field for which they are trained. To meet the estimated need of 12,000 occupational therapists, 4,000 should be graduated each year.

Of the 40,000 registered medical technologists, only 32,000 are active. Estimates of future needs vary, but even the lowest indicate that training facilities must be effectively expanded. In addition, more complex laboratory techniques require the employment of more trained technicians in several specialties, including radiological technicians, who are also in short supply.

Such programs as medical care for the aged under Social Security will undoubtedly bring about the need for a substantial increase in the supply of all types and levels of health manpower, especially social workers, to serve this age group whose social needs are frequently as great as their medical needs. The total student body in the 56 graduate schools of social work totals 6,600 students and 2,700 graduate annually.

Figures like these have become familiar to all users of health personnel. The list could be continued almost indefinitely, and all these skills are essential to personal health services. The same kinds of disparity between supply and demand exist for all types of public health personnel, in a field where new areas of activity in the broadening concern with environmental health will accentuate the shortage of personnel trained to meet modern requirements.

Determining the Scope of the Job

Before considering the methods through which an adequate supply of health personnel can be trained to do the job, it is necessary to take an honest look at what the job is. The job is to deliver quality, comprehensive health services to all citizens. Who does this? Who should do it? Wise answers are not likely to be found if we seek them only in the wilderness of the so-called population explosion. The size of the health manpower problem should not be measured solely by the size of the population, but rather by the dimensions of the actual health needs of the population — some of which, obviously, are enlarged by size. Demographic and other pertinent data are useful as guides, but health agencies should determine the personnel required to carry out their programs effectively by establishing the nature of the problems, the goals to be attained, and the number and type of personnel needed to attain these goals. [J-4]

Stretching the Manpower

Professionals involved in their own pursuits may forget that even today, when the structure of the family is changing, it would never be feasible at the going commercial rates to find enough money or personnel to provide all of the personal health services that family members give one another. Parents nurse their children, prescribe for them, and work to keep them well; the adults take care of one another, and as everyone in the family grows older, the children provide health care for their parents. Given more health education, more families can provide more and better health care in the home.

Once he leaves home to search for additional health care, the modern American of whatever social and economic status can be bedazzled, confused, and misled as he makes his choice. There are many opportunities for self-medication presented to him through every sort of communications medium. He can take himself to any one of a number of physicians, health agencies, community services, pharmacists, optometrists, podiatrists, or other licensed practitioners. He may take himself, as too many do, to a cultist or quack. The Commission believes that the individual should start with a personal physician. However, for that physician to provide the comprehensive health care that he should, he must call on the services of many allied or "helping" personnel. Many such personnel are skilled professionals in their own right and under the physician's direction are competent to provide certain aspects of health care. This brings up the necessity for proper utilization of the various kinds of health personnel, so that each "helping person" gives as much help as he is competent to give and does not waste time performing tasks that can be done as well or better by others. It is a waste of scarce health personnel if any perform tasks below the level for which they are trained, when there are others available to do such work, and dangerous for any to perform tasks beyond their respective spheres of competence.

The needs of the individual patient, the community, and every member of the health industry will be best served if each one understands the scope of his task and its relation to the tasks of those who work with him. To this end, utilization studies should be conducted to delineate the different functions required to meet the needs of patients and to determine the level of training necessary to perform these functions. [J-5] Many universities and other organizations have the resources to perform such analyses and should be supported in this effort. [I-5] This research is of immediate importance to the development of a comprehensive care program. However, certain steps to increase the efficiency of use of manpower can be taken on the basis of present information. For example, dental hygienists and other assistants with broadened functions should become a regular part of all dental practice; aides of various kinds — nursing, therapy, laboratory, clerical, and others — should be developed and used to relieve more highly skilled personnel of routine tasks; and homemakers should be trained and assigned to enlarge the effectiveness of visiting nurse services and home care programs. In addition, mental health counselors should be trained and volunteers, appropriately prepared and supervised, should be increasingly used to augment health manpower resources. Funds should be provided by both voluntary and official health agencies to test appropriate patterns for the improved use of volunteers.

These observations are made in the light of personnel changes in the past 65 years. In 1900, for every 100 physicians, there were 60 health professionals trained in other fields, including 24 dentists, 1 registered nurse, 35 pharmacists, and others trained professionally. By 1960, the relative numbers of health professionals, other than physicians, had increased so that for every 100 physicians there were 371 other professionally trained health personnel. Among the many kinds of allied health personnel are those who often work independently within the scope of their legal authority and to whom patients may come directly. These include optometrists and podiatrists. Clinical psychologists may work either independently or in cooperation with physicians and dentists and take direction and supervision for the medical or dental aspects of their work from the primary health practitioner.

The role of the nurse in coordinating orders and activities for patients from many departments of a hospital or other facility is an example of increased professional responsibility under the direction of a physician. Included in this group are pharmacists, laboratory and X-ray technicians, occupational therapists, physical therapists, dental hygienists, and many others. All of them serve two major purposes: they are supportive to the physician and allow him to treat more patients; and they increase health

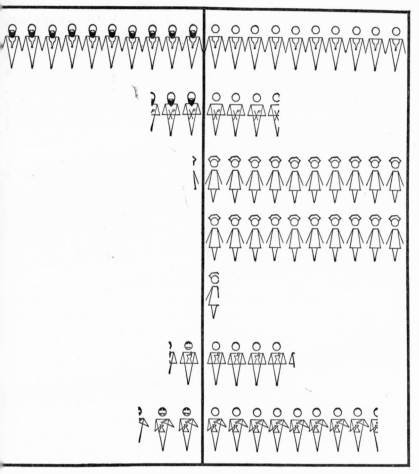

Figure 2. The proportion of physicians to allied health personnel (dentists, nurses, pharmacists, and all others), 1900 and 1960.

care efficiency because of their specialized professional competencies.

The physician is not alone in needing auxiliary help in today's complicated scientific medicine. Many of the other health professionals are in short supply, too, and effective use of their skills requires the use of differently trained personnel to extend the reach of the services they perform. More and more dentists, for example, are using assistants of various kinds, and the time has come for dental schools to assume increased responsibility for training auxiliary personnel with broadened functions and to promote their use by example. [J-6]

The use of licensed practical nurses and aides has successfully amplified nursing services. However, additional methods should be planned to aid the nurse, as her job requires more and more attention to scientific detail. The nurse needs additional clerical help to free her from the record-keeping which still takes up too much of her time in many hospitals and doctors' offices. The definition of "personnel in aid of the health professional" needs to be expanded and developed to include the auxiliary services that can be provided for social workers, therapists, and rehabilitation counselors, to mention only a few. Casework aides can help medical social workers; speech therapists can use assistants to conduct routine speech drills. In every instance, improvement in developing and assigning duties should be designed to make sure that the job is done by the person with the requisite, but minimum, training necessary to do the job.

In addition, people who have never before been considered as health workers can be involved successfully in a wide variety of "helping" situations. Community mental health and antipoverty programs, designed to meet the needs of people who have been the victims of less than adequate care, have found this different kind of worker particularly valuable. In these instances, lack of care stems in considerable part from lack of communications. The assistance of a person who shares the same background can help to reduce the effects of differences of social or economic condition, language, or other circumstances that may prevent an individual from getting the care he needs. Such a helper is known as "an indigenous nonprofessional drawn from lower socioeconomic groups."

In community action programs, the indigenous aide can perform specific and very necessary tasks by doing the legwork on which the program is based. Others can work as housing service aides, homemakers, child care aides, and parent education aides. In community health programs, they can be used as aides in home service, child service, health education, casework, and research. They possess the precious empathy too often missing among middle-class health workers and can serve a vital function as the bridge between patients or potential patients and needed health services.

A concern of a worker called "the expediter" is to activate the service relationship between agencies and clients. He gets the service and the client together and helps the client to secure the services he needs. Many a client, although accustomed to referrals and rereferrals, to long waiting lists and clinic delays, eventually becomes frustrated and despairing. The "expediter," when trained to help both his own people and the health service agencies, may well provide the missing human link that is necessary if a comprehensive health service pattern is actually to provide the continuity of care on which its concept is based.

Such nonprofessional health workers can help meet the manpower problems and make health services more effective. These developments should be further studied and applied on a broader basis.

The Commission's own experience in its Community Action Studies Project points up the need for another kind of professional health worker — the person capable of organizing and directing a community's efforts to plan for its health services. One recurrent theme in the reports of the 21 communities engaged in the Commission's work was the primacy of the Coordinator — the staff person who worked with the citizens' groups to study community needs, assess them, devise plans of action, and get the plans translated into action. Largely on the premise of these findings, the Commission recommends that schools of public health, social work, community organization, and public administration develop academic programs that will provide qualified personnel to conduct community self-studies. [J-7]

These trends toward new and wider utilization of personnel

have two basic purposes: to spread further the skills of the physician and his health care associates, and to make them more effective. The physician will continue to diagnose and outline treatment for the individual patient and he will also review the progress of the patient with other members of the health care team. Certainly, he will delegate more interim responsibility — in clearly defined areas for specified periods of time — to other health personnel. As health personnel gain more experience in this sort of community teamwork, their roles will continue to change and their training will of necessity be adapted to their new assignments. Additionally, skills such as biomedical engineering, mathematical analysis, and computer programming will become a part of the service pattern. This will not be an entirely painless process for the health professional or the health nonprofessional, but realignment of present responsibilities and roles to meet the need for a more cohesive functioning of the health team should be worth the candle, if the candle symbolizes new light by which the nation can see its way to improving the health of all people.

The Health Administrator

Modern programs of organized health care require specialized talent and training in the social and administrative sciences, as well as in the health sciences. Traditionally, the top-level administration of health services has been under the almost exclusive direction of physicians. As programs of organized health services have increased in scope and complexity, it has become increasingly clear that the years of clinical training for physicians do not necessarily equip them for the task involved. Training in administration should be available for physicians who wish to enter administrative fields.

Hospitals have pioneered in the use of nonmedical administrators. Through careful definition of administrative and clinical responsibilities, the administrator in many hospitals has been able to work in partnership with physicians to provide progressive administration of health services. In programs of community health service as well, informed, imaginative, and influential leadership by qualified administrators can achieve efficiency and fulfill the potential of these programs. Special emphasis must be given to securing and preparing top-level health service administrators for responsible positions of leadership in health. This will entail selective recruitment and training that includes administrative management, economics, sociology, and political science. Health administrators have professional satisfaction, status, and financial reward commensurate with the importance of their role. [J-8]

Environmental Health Personnel

The control of present and future environmental hazards requires personnel who are more highly specialized and better trained than in the past, and the health team of today is inadequate unless its roster includes personnel to meet all needs in this field. The public health department, as the traditional provider of public health services, has neither the personnel, the resources, the responsibility, nor the authority necessary to do an effective job of controlling today's health hazards and improving the environment of their community. Many communities are not covered by local health departments employing full-time public health officers and supporting staff. Also, many state and local health departments do not have the support, from appropriations and law enforcement procedures, needed to maintain a clean and safe community environment. This has been especially true when powerful industries, representing the nucleus around which a community maintains its economic life, have refused to cooperate with health department programs seeking the reduction or elimination of environmental pollution which they have caused.

Environmental health personnel must have a greater understanding of the relation of their work to that of other components of community life which contribute to health in its broadest sense: the relation of recreation, educational opportunity, job security, and overcrowding to individual and family health, as well as the relation to health, productivity, and length of life of the chemicals and radiation a person absorbs during his lifetime.

What is required is a reorientation of attitudes toward accepted qualifications and the exigencies of specific jobs. Most specialists in environmental health will need to be more highly trained than they are today, in view of new technological knowledge. At the same time, in some instances personnel requirements are too high for the actual work required. For example, in states requiring a sanitarian to hold a Bachelor of Science degree, the sanitarian may be more highly educated than his inspection functions require. Such personnel would be better used in supervisory and administrative capacities, aided by sanitary technicians trained to perform certain technical tasks in inspection and monitoring. In many areas of environmental health, persons with limited but specific scientific training adequate to perform well-defined tasks should be used to achieve effective and economical utilization of manpower. The United States Department of Health, Education, and Welfare should be provided with funds to support training of environmental health personnel by establishing environmental research and training centers in universities. [J-14]

As accepted procedures become routine and technical problems are conquered, the more highly trained environmental health personnel will be made available to solve new problems. For example, with supervision, technical personnel can maintain modern water-treatment plants, so that engineers and other scientists can address themselves to planning future water resources and pollution control. It is imperative that the nation find ways to use the most highly qualified professional personnel for research and experimentation with measures to control or eliminate environmental hazards.

Medical Examiners as Members of the Health Team

In addition to its other duties, an efficient medical examiner's office can also be utilized to assess a community's adequacy or lack of health care and to pinpoint the source of the inadequacy. By utilizing the knowledge it acquires from the study of the dead, the medical examiner's office helps make the community a safer and healthier place in which to live. Modern medical examiners are making important contributions to the field of vital statistics and can do more by expanding their use of computerized statistical techniques. They also assist doctors in the community to recognize areas where health care may be deficient.

Where an adequate medical examiner's law exists, the agency

is responsible for signing between 20 and 30 percent of all death certificates; where the office is scientifically operated, the quality of the vital statistics is thereby improved. Of the total deaths investigated by the medical examiner, not more than 3 or 4 percent are homicides; an approximate 10 percent are caused by vehicular accidents; and 20 percent are suicidal and accidental deaths. This means that, in the majority of cases, death was due to natural causes. Approximately half of these are sudden deaths of apparently healthy people. A great reservoir of information is available here which should be tapped to assess the causes of the deaths and perhaps point the way to prevention of similar ones in the future.

The implications of the one-half of the natural deaths certified by medical examiners where the death was not necessarily sudden, but was "unattended" by a physician, are even more significant. An epidemiologic and pathologic study of this population group in any community will provide guides to the community's medical care and indexes of its quality.

Distribution of Health Personnel

Americans are accustomed, within their own personal resources, to live and work where they want to. Economic factors may limit freedom of choice for entire segments of the population — as in parts of Appalachia — and economics are a factor in the distribution of health personnel, but, among the health professions at least, the decision to live and to practice in a given community is made principally on the basis of other factors in addition to income or salary.

Studying the distribution and use of health personnel on a national basis is made virtually impossible because of the lack of criteria defining categories of health personnel, their functions, and performance. Certainly, a detailed picture of the national distribution of health personnel is needed. Some data are available through professional organizations that take periodic surveys of their membership.

Research, teaching, and treatment facilities are of mutual benefit and tend to exist at least in a fairly close geographic proximity, if not juxtaposition. Since the location of most of the nation's universities was determined in the years prior to the recent, rapid expansion of scientific medicine, modern medical facilities are concentrated to a large extent in university communities, which in turn are usually urban centers. Because of accessibility to the latest scientific developments and expert consultation, many physicians of all specialties live and practice in these same urban centers. The same advantages that attract physicians also attract most of the other health professionals as well.

Meanwhile, many communities are without adequate health care because they have not been able to recruit personnel. Their most acute need is for personal physicians to practice in rural areas. Certain obstacles face rural communities, including isolation from the professional stimulation of frequent contact with peers facing common scientific problems and contact with colleagues engaged in research; unavailability of diagnostic tools and consultation resources to which they have become accustomed in residency training; and the absence of cultural advantages for the physician and his family.

Some communities have provided a medical student with an educational loan, in return for which the student commits himself to practice in that community for a stated period of time. The loan is made at a time when most medical students do not yet know what their intellectual and professional interests will be and the plan, therefore, has not met with great success. Some areas have acted to develop positive incentives to achieve better distribution of physicians. Such areas have created, in strategic geographic locations, modern hospitals where the medical graduate can practice scientific medicine. The Hill-Burton hospital construction program has played a significant role in such construction.

In some states, publicly financed medical care programs for the poor have provided an economic base which allows the physician to practice in an area of low socioeconomic status, where he could not possibly remain without such financing. Some states have also established clinical laboratories within the state health department with branches located in strategic areas, so that the young, well-trained physician, even in remote areas, is able to obtain most of the current microbiological, hematological, and blood chemical determinations which are essential if he is to practice the kind of medicine he has learned.

Another incentive is the establishment of a community health center or office, in which the physician practices at a low rental or lease cost. The Sears Roebuck Foundation operates a special program for this purpose. But plans of this sort will not wholly solve the problem of distribution, and it is difficult to visualize a solution at a time when personnel are in short supply and can choose their base of operation.

Recruitment

While health educators ponder the best methods of providing general health education to the public and to specific groups within the public, the health industry is only beginning to plan another kind of education — the telling of its own dynamic story in such a way that high school students, and their parents, will consider a health career as a worthwhile choice. Concerted efforts must be made to attract secondary school students to health careers by improving counseling, work experience in health facilities, and expanded work-study programs. [J-9] If the health industry hopes to secure its share of the available students, career development programs must be organized for effective competition with recruitment programs of other industries. The pioneering work of the National Health Council and state careers councils, as well as efforts of many professional associations, should be strengthened by increased financial support to make possible a continuing review of the national manpower problem and development of techniques of recruitment.

It is basic to the needs of all industries that the educational system be strengthened, and that a larger proportion of students who begin high school remain to graduate. Furthermore, more high school graduates must be accommodated in the two- and three-year colleges, to provide the technicians who will work with future professionals.

Discriminatory barriers to both education and recruitment for the health services must be removed. Civil rights legislation, federal and state antidiscrimination policies, and the work of volunteer groups are making inroads, but the nation as a whole must yet accept as fact the need to remove all discriminatory barriers to a job in any field, including health, to any qualified person whether the barrier be race, religion, age, or sex. In order to push open doors to manpower resources, governmental agencies, educational institutions, health agencies, and professional and occupational groups should undertake positive measures to recruit from part-time personnel, minority groups, the technologically displaced, and the handicapped. [J-10] Significant waste of professional manpower exists in those areas where denial of hospital staff privileges to otherwise qualified physicians on account of their race still persists. In addition, such practices have a serious adverse effect on the quality of medical care which these physicians can provide. The Commission commends those communities and institutions that have eliminated racial discrimination and segregation in the provision of health care, and urges the complete elimination of such practices in the interest of economy, good health care, and simple justice. [J-11]

Additional private and governmental funds should provide needed financial assistance for qualified and needy students at every educational level by means of scholarships, grants, and long-term loans at low interest rates. [J-14]

Teaching Community Medicine

The current undergraduate curriculum in our medical schools is divided into two main parts: the first is concentrated on anatomy, physiology, biochemistry, bacteriology, and pathology — subjects termed "the basic medical sciences." In the second part, clinical training is devoted to technical skills in diagnosis and treatment, centered on surgery, obstetrics, medicine, and pediatrics. Students receive some instruction in preventive medicine and in psychiatry, but they are not often taught social and behavioral sciences, which are basic to community medicine and psychiatry. Most of them load their premedical curriculum with the biological and chemical sciences, at the expense of learning much about the society in which they as physicians will diagnose and treat. Few educational institutions provide a young person, attracted to medicine as a social institution, the opportunity to complete his undergraduate training with special emphasis on community medicine.

Medical educators must face this question, for, no matter whether a physician devotes his time to the medical needs of individuals or to community needs, he cannot function as effectively as he might without some knowledge of the social action needed to cope with disease. As the current medical curriculum has been oriented, only after the physician has been exposed to the facts of social living, either in hospital or private practice, does he occasionally turn to community medicine as a career. It should have been possible for him to elect the study of community medicine earlier, and his curriculum could have included economics, sociology, anthropology, and epidemiology as well as clinical instruction.

From this type of curriculum, the student could select a career as a personal physician, working directly with patients and their families; he could choose occupational health; or he could choose to concern himself with the means for providing comprehensive health care to all the individuals in the community, rather than with the direct provision of care. From this type of medical curriculum could come the young physician trained to accept some of the profession's emerging responsibilities to the community. He could be trained to direct the many activities involved in modern community medicine — activities related to professional and allied health personnel, facilities, financial resources, and institutions responsible for the provision of community health.

The university medical centers should accept their responsibility to provide an adequate research and educational framework to prepare the physician for his new role in society. Graduate schools of public health, business administration, and public administration should extend their training of professional health or medical care administrators.

There are times in man's history when teaching has progressed quietly and dogmatically, and has dealt more with technology than with concept; at other times, the whole teaching process catches fire. Men honored from that time on transmit the excitement to their students, and the students enter their careers prepared not only to earn a good life for themselves, but to show the way toward a good life for other men. We are ready for such a time in the teaching of all the health professions, the technicians, and the aides.

Other Training Needs: Social Workers

A new look at the curriculum of the medical school may well serve as the key to providing physicians adequately trained for modern medical practice. But this is only the foundation; additional funds and teaching resources are needed in other disciplines as well. The shortage of trained social workers, for example, is one of the most acute in the health field, and is destined to become even more so as more people over 65 are able to finance health care. Vigorous efforts, voluntary and governmental, must be undertaken to increase the supply of professional social workers in medical and health services through the construction of expanded and new educational facilities; financial support for faculty field instructors and related costs of teachers; greatly increased scholarship aid through fellowships and traineeships; and research and experimentation in methods of professional education aimed at innovations intended to improve the quality of professional education of social workers for medical and health services. [J-12]

There should be increased training for social workers in medical and health settings, where training is community-oriented and provided in concert with other members of the health team. In addition, since it is probable that graduate schools are not going to produce enough social workers to meet the increasing needs in this field, research and demonstration must proceed toward a teaching program to train personnel of less than professional skills to perform limited duties within the health team. [J-13]

Additional financing is needed not only for students of social work; all qualified candidates for training in a health career should receive the financial assistance they need from government, industry, or other sources, in the form of grants, scholarships or loans, to complete their training. [J-14]

Nursing Programs

Eighty percent of our registered nurses are graduated from the three-year diploma schools of nursing. These institutions are a proven source of supply and deserve support.

Efforts must be intensified to expand accredited nursing education programs which prepare persons to become registered nurses with college degrees through baccalaureate programs; registered nurses without college degrees through two-year colleges or hospital diploma programs; and vocational or practical nurses through vocational school or hospital programs. [J-15]

The expansion and quality of these educational programs are dependent upon the necessary number of qualified teachers, administrators, and clinically expert nurses who assume responsibility for the educational program and the clinical practice through which students are introduced to comprehensive patient care. There is imperative need for a sufficient number of registered nurses graduated from baccalaureate programs, which is the entree to the graduate programs through which teachers, administrative personnel, and specialized clinical practitioners receive their formal nursing education.

Two-Year Colleges

Since the two-year community colleges can play an important role in training auxiliary health personnel, present programs for health occupations in junior colleges should be expanded as rapidly as is consistent with quality. Curriculums in two-year colleges should be designed, insofar as possible, to permit additional education at a later time for those students who want to continue their health career development. Two-year colleges should be aided by: grants from private sources and government to develop training programs for health occupations; federal funds to universities for the preparation of faculty required to teach in two-year colleges; scholarships from private and government funds to students in two-year colleges who wish to prepare for health occupations; affiliation with four-year colleges and medical institutions that can supply laboratory and clinic experience, as well as consultation and association with health professionals. [J-16]

In the establishment of more health curriculums in the two-year colleges, administrators and faculties will need help from universities, professional schools, and health agencies in the area. Health programs in the two-year colleges should be planned on a state and regional level. They should be developed in close functional relation to health service organizations and to institutions of higher education. Affiliation should be maintained with a medical center, hospital, or other health facility. With proper planning and development, health programs in these colleges can serve the immediate needs of community health services for auxiliary personnel of many kinds and can also direct certain students toward the goal of further education. The development and execution of such a program of education for the health occupations in the two-year college is a challenge that will undoubtedly present difficulties, but the reward will be increased numbers of well-trained health service personnel.

The growth of two-year colleges provides a new potential source of health personnel. It is possible that within the next few years, the nation as a whole may accept the idea and achieve the goal of extending public education to include vocational and technical schools, junior colleges, and the first two years of the four-year college, so that a student has the opportunity to participate in 14 years of publicly supported education. The Commission's Task Force on Manpower reports the present health education picture both in depth and breadth. It is not enough to train more people in the same old way; health training must initiate change, so that personnel, upon graduation, will be equipped to meet the newly forming dimensions of jobs in health care.

Education: The Team Approach, Standards

To the fullest extent possible, members of the health team should receive their education jointly in order to give each an appreciation of the goals and skills of the other, plus practical experience in working together on common problems. [J-17] Education for the health professions and their coworkers at all levels must be strengthened. Only by redesigning education so that individuals of all health disciplines train together as students, in the same fashion that they will work together after graduation, can this nation substitute action for talk.

The standards of schools offering training to various kinds of technicians needed in modern health services must be universally established and enforced. The field of education of technicians, perhaps because it is newer than that of professional education, demands immediate attention if the public is to be protected and assured of high and uniform quality. Current programs of education in the health field, like available health services, range from quackery to superb presentations by distinguished faculties. The student needs aid in selecting his education, just as the patient needs assistance in getting the services he needs; and the student must be assured that the training he selects prepares him adequately for his work.

Continuing Education

While recruiting individuals into health services and concerning itself with the education of young people as they enter the field, the health industry must simultaneously concentrate on means to provide continuing education for the people who are now at work. Educational institutions offering health training should cooperate actively with professional associations and official and private agencies in developing programs of in-service training and continuing education for allied health services personnel. [J-18]

Leadership institutes are useful tools for training health service personnel in the concepts of community planning and action. In addition, there should be a wide variety of educational programs that can give in-service, or on-the-job training to all levels of health personnel. Such in-service programs, of course, exist today. They must be strengthened in order that men and women now at work, and the young graduates who will join them shortly, can progressively increase their skills and accept larger responsibilities.

One example of an effective in-service training program is that administered by the National Institute of Mental Health — financed by matching federal and state grants — in which state mental hospitals and institutions for the mentally retarded are upgrading the skills of their nonprofessional workers. Since these are the workers who are in daily contact with their patients and provide most of the routine care, such a program might serve as a model for other health facilities within the community.

At the professional level, the medical specialty of pathology, through its professional organization, the American Society of Clinical Pathologists, conducts a continuing education program which, since its inception in 1958, has consisted of a series of regional workshops and tutorials and has always been oversubscribed. In addition, the association presents a monthly Check Sample program, through which pathologists are mailed "unknowns" in the categories of chemistry, pathology, hematology, immunity, microbiology, and special topics of interest. They and their laboratory technicians test the samples together and in so doing improve their competences. By 1970, it is anticipated that 5,000 pathologists will be involved in the program and that it will require preparation and distribution of approximately 95,000 "unknown" specimens. These programs are entirely financed within the specialist's organization. Other medical groups present other types of programs designed to keep their members abreast of current knowledge.

Based on past performance, the Commission is confident that the United States can provide an adequate supply of health manpower if, along with creating new systems, we remodel the traditional approaches to solution of the manpower problems in the various health and medical fields of activity — but both pride and prejudice will be shaken before that job is done.

CHAPTER VI

The Places for Personal Health Care

When a community actually goes to work to establish a comprehensive system of personal health care for all its residents, it must obtain certain kinds of information. First, it needs to know who the potential consumers of health care are — their groups, social and economic characteristics; next, it must know the composition of its skilled supply of health manpower and its work habits; and then, the community must take a long, hard look at the places that are providing services on which people rely for personal health care. These places comprise an industry of tremendous size and scope. They encompass: the hospital, in its most comprehensive sense, including extended care facilities and home care programs; related health care facilities, such as personal care and residential centers; community health programs, public and voluntary; and personal services of physicians and other health professionals. All of these need to be known in terms of their quality and variety, as well as number.

When almost any community holds the mirror of a self-study up to its health services, it usually discovers that one place — one facility — has the center of the stage for patient care: the hospital. How the responsibility of a hospital is conceived for comprehensive personal health care, and how the hospital thus develops its services to deliver both the in-hospital and the out-of-hospital care available and accessible to all the people will determine whether or not other facilities and services will be established effectively — that is, in the home, in extended care facilities, and in more specialized centers. The community's general hospitals increasingly are broadening the scope of their activities beyond their four walls, and in so doing are more and more taking on a role in coordinating broader community health services and facilities. In fact, changing concepts and characteristics of hospital utilization are pointing to the hospital — a dynamic operation involving governing board, medical staff, and administration — as a center for community health services or the locus of a community health campus.

The integration of health care agencies can be assisted by geographical proximity, each maintaining operating independence but having a more workable opportunity to cooperate for the benefit of patients and agencies. Some communities, looking to coordinating present services and filling future needs, are experimenting with the "health campus" approach. Such a campus groups certain community health care facilities and services: the official health department, offices of voluntary health associations, offices for physicians, laboratories, extended care facilities, nursing homes, rehabilitation centers, mental health centers, and, of course, the hospital. Even though geographic proximity is not always possible, nevertheless, functional coordination is imperative. This concept applies not only in urban centers, but also in rural areas, even for the physician's office. "Satellite" hospitals or medical centers are particularly suited for rural areas.

Advocates of the campus concept point to the ease with which patients can get from needed service to needed service and the ease with which physicians and allied health personnel can move from the patient in the hospital to the one in the nursing home or the rehabilitation center. Others counter with the increased difficulty the family of the patient may have in visiting him or taking over part of his care. If an aunt is in a nursing home near her nieces and nephews, she is likely to get a great deal more attention and help than if she is several miles and bus transfers away. To enhance the quality of care they provide, health campuses and other forms of community organization of facilities and services need to encourage constant experimentation and innovation.

The Hospital

In the practice of modern scientific medicine, the physician depends increasingly upon associated services. The material, facilities, and technical personnel required for the diagnosis and treatment of disease have increased substantially; as a result the capital investment and operating costs for providing medical services have been enlarged beyond the means of most individual physicians to supply. But to prevent illness, to save and extend human life, there must be a converging of the diverse, highly specialized human skills and mechanical devices, so that the correlation and synthesis of knowledge essential to quality medical care can be achieved.

The hospital is the converging point for many of these skills and specialized equipment. It is here that many physician specialists, nurses, pharmacists, social workers, therapeutic dieticians, laboratory and X-ray technologists, physical and occupational therapists, medical record librarians, and scores of other specialized workers unite their skills with mechanical devices in their common purpose to preserve and restore health.

While presently many medical services may be scattered all over the lot, figuratively as well as actually, it is the opinion of many that the effective correlation of related but separate medical units in a community can best be secured through development of a program of health care based upon the hospital as the core of the medical complex. If this is to occur, the hospitals themselves must take the lead in changing their own attitudes.

Surveys and reports indicate that hospitals in many communities have tended to operate in splendid isolation, perhaps because they saw themselves as self-sufficient in the medical talent and the mechanical technology necessary to serve most of the needs of most patients. This attitude is changing dramatically, and, if the hospital continues to look outside its windows into the doors of other agencies, it can become the facility, the place of reference for much of a community's medical service. Viewed in this light, the future general hospital, providing comprehensive medical services in the acute, chronic, and psychiatric fields, while emphasizing prevention, care, and rehabilitation, can become an integrating factor in community health care facilities.

The hospital represents the common ground of medical care on which the patient, community, and professional groups can meet. It provides many of the needed specialized and expensive facilities. It occupies a strategic position in the community to coordinate various health activities, both voluntary and public. Because the central hospital and its satellites provide the equipment and auxiliary personnel needed by the personal physician, the availability of its services to more sparsely populated areas can become a significant force to encourage physicians to locate their practices outside the major metropolitan areas. In Manitoba, Canada, and elsewhere, it has been demonstrated that the hospital outside the major metropolitan area attracts physicians to locate in its vicinity.

These are general statements arising out of the Commission's work. During the same period, other studies have expressed more specific points of view on this subject. The report of an ad hoc subcommittee of the State of Maryland Commission to Study Hospital Costs presents a forthright commentary on what could be expected of today's hospital by its community. This *Report to the Governor* (1964, p. 109) indicates needed changes and trends that should be developed. The subcommittee was composed of women whose occupations ranged from housewife to business woman, school principal, and social worker. Although none of them was closely connected with a general hospital, other than through work in a hospital auxiliary, most had had a member of the immediate family as a hospital patient within two years prior to the study. The report reflects a sophisticated consumer point of view, expressed by a group of women deeply concerned with the health of their families.

This group expected the hospital to serve as the focus for all medical care services. The hospital, the report stated, could provide the security for the consumer of being able to reach medical help quickly. The group recommended that hospitals provide a wide range of hospital-based services, including increased, round-the-clock emergency services and more involvement in a total rehabilitative program. They recognized the interrelation of social and physical needs. They brought out also that overuse of the hospital cannot be entirely identified by applying medical criteria alone to a human situation. The report expressed the hope that there would be more coordination of medical and social needs of outpatients, and that coordination between hospital and nursing homes would be closer.

It was apparent that this group of women looked to the hospital with its accessibility, availability of professional talent, and readiness to serve, as a substitute for the remembered — if perhaps idealized — comforting reassurance and availability of the old-time family doctor, who worked in a less complicated society. This attitude was emphasized by the request that the hospital staff be more friendly and take the time to explain treatment processes to the patient and his family. The medical profession, the group said, both inside and outside the hospital, should take time to enlighten patients. In summary, the committee agreed that the hospital should be the place where the patient can rely upon medical knowledge, skills, and services, given in an understanding manner and available at any time of day or night.

Can the Hospital Do It All?

Can a hospital meet all needs and provide all services? Should it? The report of the State of New York Governor's Committee on Hospital Costs (*Summary of Findings and Recommendations,* April 9, 1965), an extensive and useful survey of hospital services, addresses itself to these questions. The committee recommended that a hospital affiliate itself with other facilities designed to provide specific types of care. It concluded that the cost of patient care can be reduced if patients are treated in facilities most appropriate to their needs, if the proper degree of care is given for the correct amount of time, and if drugs and other medications are provided at minimal cost consistent with high quality. In that case, hospitals would be used primarily for patients with conditions not treatable outside the hospital. Following this course would bring up the necessity for a constellation of medical services. Many communities lack such services in adequate supply and quality.

If a patient cannot find another place in which to be treated, or if his prepaid insurance is limited to care provided in a hospital, then he and his physician turn to the hospital — where care is most expensive — even if hospitalization is not really needed. In the progress of many illnesses, hospital care is necessary only in the acute period, but if no alternate facilities are available, the patient's stay in the hospital is extended and the costs go up, for himself, the community, and those who share the cost of his prepayment insurance. Organized home care programs like those discussed in Chapter II are a useful device to remove the burden of extended care from the general hospital. There are others as well. High priority must be given to the development, in the hospital or affiliated with the hospital, of extended care facilities, self-care units, rehabilitation units, home care programs, geriatric day centers, foster family programs, and outpatient services to provide a network of alternative services and to encourage appropriate utilization of facilities. [K-1]

Hospital Management

It is undoubtedly true that no community will be successful in establishing an integrated pattern of medical services, imaginatively and economically administered, until its hospitals are functioning with optimal effectiveness. The lines of organization within the hospital are clear. The board of trustees has the ultimate authority; the medical staff and the administration each has its own, subject to the board. The clear definition of these responsibilities has been developed over the years to correspond with the increasing complexity of the modern hospital, although there are still individual institutions in which the lines of authority are ill-defined or overlapping. It is important that the medical staff be involved with organizational matters related to its area of authority; that the board of trustees distinguish between matters of policy and matters of management, and restrict its authority to decisions of policy; and that the administration utilize every tool available to it to achieve effective management. To the extent that the triad of authority is not fulfilling its responsibilities, is not clearly defined, or is not functioning harmoniously, the hospital cannot be optimally effective.

Members of the medical staff in most hospitals should be further integrated into the hospital's administration, since the physician's decisions relate to every facet of the hospital's operation. As the American Hospital Association has said (in *The*

Changing Hospital and the American Hospital Association, 1965, p. 5): "The physician is no longer merely a welcome and essential 'visiting man' on the hospital stage. He is increasingly involved in the organizational workings of the hospital. He must be given the opportunity and the responsibility to help write the organizational script as well as act from it. The hospital medical staff is becoming increasingly the organizational center of the professional activities of the whole medical care system in a community."

Individual medical staff members have at times been slow to consider needs other than those of their own patients and their personal practice. The physician, however, is the man who decides who shall enter the hospital, at what time he shall enter (subject to the availability of beds), how long he shall remain, and what tests, medications, and other treatments shall be provided. Some physicians order more tests than others; physicians in solo practice may use the hospital in ways that differ from those of physicians practicing in groups. Not enough physicians consider the value of collaborating with other members of the medical staff in scheduling their vacations in order that the hospital can strive for maximum utilization throughout the year; most surgeons prefer to operate in the morning, and very few prefer to use the surgery on Saturdays and Sundays, except in emergencies. Concerted action on the part of physicians on hospital staffs will be necessary if the hospital's services are to be utilized more successfully. This can be achieved through the organized medical staff with its various department heads and established committees. Through this administrative construction, attention can be given to such matters as the appropriateness of utilization of facilities and services and means of avoiding peaks and valleys in occupancy and in the use of special services.

Hospitals and doctors can achieve closer relationships in making fuller use of the hospital's diagnostic and therapeutic services for ambulatory patients. Appropriate outpatient department arrangements would encourage more frequent use of these services by the walk-in patient, reporting for tests or treatments at his physician's prescription.

The importance of the physician in determining length of stay, and the variation among physicians in this respect, has been pointed out. According to a University of Michigan study of hospital and medical economics,* general practitioners tend to discharge patients too soon more often than do board-certified specialists, while the specialists tend to keep their patients in the hospital for an unnecessary length of time. However, many factors other than individual practices or local custom are involved in length of stay, including such things as population characteristics, morbidity rates, utilization rates, number of hospital beds and alternative facilities per 1000 population, capital investment in health facilities and the sources of such investment, per capita income, extent of prepayment coverage, and comprehensiveness of services provided.

It is imperative, then, for the medical staff to become more closely related to the hospital administration, for, even though the physician's overriding responsibility is to provide the highest possible quality of care for his patients, he must also — in this period of rising costs and public demand for efficient administration — share the responsibility for providing that care efficiently and economically. No longer can the physician expect to continue in the old ways; he not only practices medicine within the hospital; he must accept the fact that he is a part of the hospital, even though he is not employed by the institution. In 1966, the staff privilege accorded a physician by a hospital carried with it the acceptance of a responsibility as a working member of an organized staff structure functioning administratively through department heads.

In the same fashion, the hospital board of trustees must be evaluated in the community frame of reference. Boards of trustees have in large measure been made up of dedicated and knowledgeable people, but the modern hospital is a very complex institution; few industries would appoint a board of directors today on the basis that many hospital boards have been assembled in the past. As has been traditional in philanthropic organizations, many hospital board members are still appointed because of their personal philanthropy to the hospital, or their social or

---

* Walter J. McNerney *et al., Hospital and Medical Economics: A Study of Population, Service, Costs, Methods of Payment, and Controls,* 2 vols., Chicago: Hospital Research and Educational Trust, 1962.

power position in the community, although hospital philanthropy has become increasingly directed to the area of capital financing and research, rather than the subsidy of deficits. Reimbursement for operating costs has become largely the responsibility of the individual patient, prepayment, and government. When such appointments are predominant, the board will tend to have a parochial interest in one institution, a limited knowledge of the social forces pressing upon health facilities to adapt their services to common need, and as a result a reluctance to take a bold new look at the hospital's place in the health service community. If private nonprofit hospitals are to become the nuclei for community health services, hospital board members must be selected from persons who are aware of the total health needs of the community, and the means by which the specific hospital whose policies they are responsible for setting can best fit into a community pattern. Trustees of hospitals must add sophisticated knowledge to their good works if a comprehensive service pattern is to become a reality. To help them, there should be established, within the framework of regional or state hospital associations, groups — composed of trustees, medical staff, and administrators — that could promote a broader outlook, and serve as information sources and forums for the exchange of ideas. [K-2]

In the past the hospital administrator has often been hampered by board interference in matters of management, rather than aided by board direction in matters of policy. In earlier days, when hospitals were simpler and administrative matters less specialized and complex, hospital trustees participated rather frequently in hospital business or administrative matters of special interest to them, especially in the smaller hospitals. As hospitals grew in size and in complexity, the areas of responsibility of the board, medical staff, and administration became more clearly defined. The fact that hospital administration had become a specialty of business administration was demonstrated when the first graduate program in hospital administration was established at the University of Chicago Graduate School of Business in 1934.

Opportunities to educate administrative personnel for hospital posts must be expanded, and two aspects of that education emphasized. Those responsible for the education of hospital administrators must emphasize that understanding the health community of which the hospital is a part and relating the hospital effectively to allied health care facilities and programs are basic to success as an effective administrator. [K-3] Such knowledge will open up to the hospital administrator possible sources of help with the problems of his own hospital, and break down the hedges of self-containment that have been allowed to grow around most hospitals. The modern hospital administrator also needs to be at home in the world of data processing, budgets, and operational research. Hospitals and allied facilities should explore every available additional means for improving management, increasing efficiency, and reducing cost. Such means should include systems of joint management — laundries, laboratories, drug formularies, and purchasing services — and exploration of the possibility of merging small hospitals. [K-4] Administrators should take advantage of the programs now available by which these objectives can be accomplished. Examples are three American Hospital Association programs: The Management Review Program; Hospital Administrative Services; and the Manpower for Health Program.

Hospital trustees must provide funds with which administrators can establish procedures for refined cost analysis, job analysis, supervisory training of employees, and budgetary planning that relate to those used in other facilities in a given community. With modern cost accounting, computerized data processing, and, more importantly, a clear line of authority in relation to the trustees and the medical staff, the hospital administrator can and must expedite the effective delivery of health care. It will become more feasible, as the health facilities utilize modern administrative techniques, for several of them to assume joint responsibility for the cost and operation of such techniques as well as for laboratory and computer programs and drug formularies. It will be advantageous for all health care facilities in a community to secure technical assistance to help them establish administrative procedures capable of maintaining the steady flow of services in all facilities on an effectively organized and economical routine program.

The Cost of Hospital Care

The public has indicated repeatedly that it will pay for high quality health care, but since hospital costs have continued to rise across the country, there is a growing public insistence that everything possible be done to avoid unnecessary increases in cost and to eliminate waste and duplication.

The rapid rise in the cost of hospital care in the past two decades is a matter of grave concern to the American people. The cost has continued steadily to increase at the rate of 6.5 percent a year. At this rate, hospital costs double every ten to eleven years. Only with continued improvements in management and efficiency can the rate of increase be held in check. The upward pressure on costs results from the development of new and costlier diagnostic and treatment techniques; increases in salary costs as hospital wages become competitive with industry; additional personnel to man new or expanded services, compensate for reductions in the work week, and provide more hours of coverage; the increasing burden of educational and training programs in hospitals; and the inability of hospitals to match rising costs with increased productivity.

The Commission takes the position that further increases in hospital costs must not be accepted complacently, but that a wide range of vigorous and persistent actions must be taken by all parties concerned to moderate the costs of hospital care without adverse effects on its quality. [K]

Research and demonstration grants to hospitals, councils, universities, and other organizations to support studies of hospital operating costs and capital financing, as well as pioneering programs aimed at cost reduction, are a manifest need. [K-5] Grant support should be made available to help the community retool its health facilities into a cohesive and coordinated system. The entire community stands to benefit if hospital costs can be reduced by measures to improve the efficiency of the delivery of health services. These measures would include eliminating unnecessary duplication and waste, changing financing procedures so that the individual patient does not pay for those hospital services — such as emergency services — that are provided to serve the entire community, and expanding insurance coverage to include more services. A wide variety of existing conditions will affect progress in this direction. It would be so much easier if a community could start from the beginning.

In some areas, there are too many hospitals. Although they are becoming fewer, there remain today some hospitals that should never have been built, as and where they are, and there are hospitals that should no longer be operated. One of the unfortunate results of this situation is that skilled health personnel is concentrated too heavily in some areas, is not used for maximum efficiency, and has no interest in practicing in other areas in which hospital facilities are desperately needed.

No hospital can be expected to maintain 100 percent occupancy at all times; indeed, optimum occupancy is 85 to 90 percent, since the hospital must have approximately 10 percent of its beds empty to provide for turnover. But empty beds are expensive beds; one estimate places the cost of an empty bed at three-fourths the cost of an occupied bed. This is a problem that defies complete solution. There are too many beds in maternity and pediatric departments of hospitals in many instances, and a severe national shortage of chronic hospital and nursing home beds. To provide for the efficient utilization of all hospitals in a community, every health service would have to agree to close down or replace institutions that are obsolete for any reason; to convert others to new uses; to consolidate others and coordinate their programs; and, if new facilities are needed, to build them so that they can be adapted to the changing needs of a changing patient population.

Establishing a community health care facilities system of this sort within a community will take legislation in some instances; it will require the surrender, in others, of autonomy carefully preserved by individual hospital boards over the years. It will also change the usual highly competitive attitudes of hospitals in some communities where it is generally accepted that each hospital should provide all facilities and services, no matter how rarely a community needs them: for example, facilities for open heart surgery and high energy radiation. Many reasons lie behind hospital improvement or expansion of medical services, among them the needs of the medical staffs and educational programs and the requirements of the accrediting agencies. These reasons will continue to exist. The change that must come, then, is a change in the entire attitude toward increased services. Instead of acting alone, hospital facilities must plan and act in concert. The emerging trend in this direction was exemplified late in 1965 by the establishment of the Wilmington, Delaware, Medical Center. This center resulted from the merger of three hospitals under one unified board, with medical care provided by one unified medical staff and management by one unified administration although all three hospital plants were still in operation. The objectives of the merger were not only to achieve improvement of operation and utilization but also to enhance the excellence of medical care for the community as a whole.

To assure the best utilization of manpower and money, hospital and related health facility planning must be both regional and rational. Such planning — especially when it deals with matters of capital expenditure — must be based on identified need, supported by reliable factual information. New facilities in any community should be built for one reason only: proven need. If the development of comprehensive personal health care, provided with continuity in the community, is to become a reality, it is crucial that the relation between health facility planning and health services planning be both recognized and honored. Regional health planning councils (discussed in Chapter VII) should be responsible for initiating or coordinating health facility planning for the region. For health facility planning to be effective, the responsible planning group should be provided with sufficient authority to assure coordination of equipment, space, staff, and utilization of facilities within its jurisdictions as well as authority to review and evalute plans for new facility construction or change of function. [K-6]

Paid in Full

Many philanthropic and governmental agencies do not now pay the full cost for services rendered to their patients. The effort to obtain full reimbursement and the development of equitable bases for payment has involved hospitals and many organizations and agencies for many years. Notable achievements have been the development of reimbursable cost formulas, pioneered in the 1940's, and their adoption by a majority of Blue Cross plans and many governmental agencies; the American Hospital Association's Principles of Payment for Hospital Care; and, in 1965, the acceptance of "reasonable cost" as a basis for payment under Medicare. Unfortunately, some agencies which supposedly base reimbursement on costs restrict their payment by imposing an arbitrary maximum or ceiling. The difference in what these agencies pay and what the services actually cost must then be absorbed by the hospital — that is, added to other patients' bills — or loss of income affects the hospital's ability to provide comprehensive, high quality services. The Commission concurs with its Task Force on Financing Community Health Services and Facilities in recommending that third parties — health insurance plans and governmental agencies — pay the hospital for services rendered at full current cost. [K-7] In turn, the hospital is expected to exert every effort to collect its bills. Income from philanthropy can help defray the cost of care rendered to the medically indigent. The remainder of the cost should be met through a pro rata allocation to all patients. As more and more hospital care moves into the pattern of full payment, it will be important for payment plans to incorporate devices to encourage reduction in cost and reward efficiency of operation. Further study is needed in this area.

Education Costs Money

Hospitals have for many years been the primary source of training for a major portion of health personnel — nurses, interns, residents, and many kinds of allied personnel. In 1965, the extent of this program annually included about 100,000 students in training to be registered nurses, with about 900 hospitals involved; over 20,000 students of practical nursing, involving over 300 hospitals; nearly 10,000 physicians in internship programs, involving over 850 hospitals; plus thousands of students, interns, and residents in health specialties such as medical technology, dietetics, hospital administration, and medical records administration. The costs of educating these vitally necessary personnel should not be borne by the patients who happen to be confined to the hospital during the time these workers are being trained. Research must be undertaken to determine the net cost of educating interns, residents, medical students, nurses, and other allied professional and technical personnel, and to determine the appropriate sources of funds for meeting those costs. [K-8]

Different patterns are possible and appropriate: one hospital may wish to retain its entire education and training program with support from the educational system in the community or state. Others may wish gradually to divest themselves of one or more aspects of their education programs and assist a neighboring two-year college in taking it over. The Commission does not intend to recommend the methods health facilities use to accomplish the goal; it is concerned only that the cost of educating health personnel not be handed on to the individual patient.

The same argument is persuasive for other services often rendered by the health facility services that are maintained for the community at large. For example, the difference between what it costs to maintain an emergency room or ambulance service and what the hospital or other health facility is able to collect from users of that service should be borne by philanthropy and the community at large — not by the cancer patient on 3B whose bill is already a matter of concern to his family and his insurance company.

Utilization of Health Facilities

As anyone who has ever been a patient in a modern hospital knows, in anything but exceptional circumstances, to enter a hospital on Friday is to spend a lost weekend. It is claimed by some that one of the simplest methods of putting a hospital to better use would be to put it on a 7-day, 24-hour total working basis. True, hospitals do operate every day of every year, but the operation on weekends and during most of the night are on a custodial basis, for the most part. Laboratories, surgeries, and examination rooms are usually dark, except for the standard 40-hour week.

The New York Governor's Committee on Hospital Costs reported that, on any given day, at least 10 percent of the patients in general hospitals did not need to be there. Tests are necessary in many potential hospital cases, but often the only reason that the patient is admitted to the hospital for testing, rather than walking in to be tested and returning home to await the results, is the fact that such tests are not covered by his hospital benefits unless he is admitted to the hospital. At the other end of the illness cycle — the period of convalescence or rehabilitation — many patients remain in the hospital, using and paying for the full hospital care facilities, when they could either continue treatment as an outpatient, or take care of most of their needs, while in the hospital, on their own initiative. Many hospitals have added self-care units with good results. Self-care cuts costs and also helps the patient toward self-confidence and total recovery. Communities must experiment with pilot projects and demonstrations to test specific procedures to achieve maximum efficient use of facilities. [K-9]

Extended Care Facilities

The widest gap in health care facilities in most parts of the United States today is the lack of sufficient places to meet the long-term illness requirements of the increasing numbers of older persons in our society — acceptable beds in nursing homes, progressive patient care approaches in general hospitals, infirmary units in homes for the aged.

More and more people who are chronically ill cannot be cared for in their homes. Three-generation households are no longer the rule in the United States. Apartment living, economic considerations, lack of domestic help, and other factors have severely limited the ability of the family unit of 1966 to provide residential care for illnesses other than those that occur and run their course in a brief period of time. The construction of extended care facilities under voluntary nonprofit auspices physically or functionally related to a general hospital is a top priority. [K-10] High quality chronic care units can be operated as part of the hospital at 30 to 50 percent less than the cost of acute hospital care. It will also help to alleviate the shortage of available facilities for the chronically ill if nursing homes, even though independent of the hospital administration, are linked to the hospital through an organized outpatient system, and are utilized by the hospital, as it assumes responsibility to transfer a patient who no longer needs acute hospital care to an appropriate treatment setting. To make such a system effective, of course, prepayment and insurance benefits for extended care must be expanded.

Community Mental Health Centers

Because of the neglect of facilities for the promotion of mental health and the treatment of mental illness, the Commission has chosen to emphasize this area of needed services, with no intent to diminish the importance of all other types of facilities. For more than 100 years, Americans have become so accustomed to placing the major responsibility for providing care for the mentally ill and mentally retarded upon the state that even health professionals, generally, do not consider the state mental hospital a part of the community health system. Because of advances in treatment techniques, increasing numbers of general hospitals are admitting mental patients for short-term, intensive treatment. It is significant that half the total number of hospital beds in the country are occupied by mentally ill patients.

The future looks much brighter for the emotionally disturbed or mentally ill patient, but no century-old system of care can be changed in a few months. Hospital boards of trustees, medical staffs, and administrators have been slow to realize, as have the governmental authorities, that the cost of caring for the mentally ill is also a cost assumed by the community, even though it has in some ways been a "hidden cost," within the state or county tax structure.

Important new concepts are now working to bring treatment for the mentally ill back into the mainstream of American medicine and into the comprehensive community-based program of health services. One of these is the establishment of community mental health centers. The development and administration of these centers are being devised in a number of ways. The intent is to utilize the existing resources of a community first, and to construct new facilities when they are needed to provide one or more of the essential elements of care required to treat the mentally ill. High priority for both construction and staffing funds for community mental health centers is accorded those centers that include a general hospital in the grouping of facilities.

In order to meet the needs of the mental patient, it is imperative that there are easily available resources for diagnosis. This can be provided by the personal physician if he has been trained to recognize all, and treat the less severe, psychiatric disturbances. Diagnosis of the more complex case is made by the psychiatrist. In many instances, others, although not equipped to treat emotional illness, are able to recognize symptomatic behavior which signals the need for such treatment.

Utilizing modern therapies, it is often unnecessary for a mental patient to be hospitalized on a 24-hour basis, and, if hospitalization is prescribed, it can be of short duration. Some hospitals operate separate psychiatric units; others treat mental patients in the general service; still others maintain psychiatric outpatient clinics. Some mental patients, although they do not need full-time hospitalization, do need day or night hospital care. To meet this need, hospitals are providing partial hospitalization, for example, for the person who can be maintained at school or on the job during the day, but needs counseling, therapy, and custodial care at night. Others, who may be able to remain at home at night, need the support of treatment and rehabilitation during the day.

If it is difficult in modern society to locate a doctor in the middle of the night for a house call, it is immeasurably more difficult to find help when a psychiatric crisis occurs. Then, too, mental illness still retains legal and protective overtones which often produce traumatic experiences for the patient. Psychiatric emergency services must be provided as part of every community health service pattern. No longer should the uniformed policeman be the person who answers the call for emergency help and no longer should the jail be the place to which the mentally ill are taken in crises.

If general hospitals today are not utilized efficiently at night and on weekends for physical illness, they are even more remiss in providing psychiatric service at these times. In a few communities, as many as 72 hours can elapse before the court procedures necessary to certify a mental patient for treatment can occur; during that time, under the current statutes, medical personnel are not allowed to treat the patient. Such appalling conditions can be reversed in communities that organize and operate a community mental health center providing as essential care inpatient service, day and night hospital service, outpatient service, emergency service, and consultative and educational services designed to integrate care of the mentally ill into the community by working with all the community agencies concerned. Preadmission care, aftercare, and rehabilitation are as vitally a part of modern treatment for the mentally ill as for those whose illnesses are primarily physical, and these services can be integrated within one community plan.

It is not necessary that all services provided by a community mental health center be available under one roof, or even under one administrative entity. Various types of agreements have been devised through which a group of independently administered facilities — a general hospital, an outpatient clinic, a university center, and a publicly financed day care unit, for example — can affiliate to provide comprehensive psychiatric care and qualify for federal grants-in-aid. The comprehensive community mental health centers plan is already under way in some locations. It is important that, as these centers develop, they do so as part of the total health services system, both for the provision of better care to the patient and because modern medical knowledge must be utilized in concert with new knowledge about man's behavior and the effects of his environment on his health, if he is to receive the highest quality of treatment.

One of the steps that must be taken if the integration of psychiatric with other medical treatment is to be achieved can be worked out only by the medical profession. There is growing realization that all qualified physicians in a community should be accorded appropriate staff privileges in patient care facilities within that community. This is especially necessary in terms of treatment of mental illness. If, for example, the personal physician diagnoses a psychiatric disorder which is beyond his competence to treat, he can hospitalize his patient in a psychiatric service within the hospital, or refer him to a psychiatrist, in the same manner that he refers patients to other medical specialists. In either case it is considered important today for the personal physician to maintain contact with his patient, in order to provide better care following the acute phase of illness; his doing so can markedly influence the patient's recovery.

This will mean, if a general hospital is to operate as a part of a community mental health center, that appropriate staff privileges must be accorded to all qualified physicians who request them. As more hospital administrators and physicians become accustomed to the need for collaboration among hospitals, rather than competition, this procedure will undoubtedly be accelerated, but at present it is one of the blocks to community-wide use of all health services.

Utilization of the Mental Hospital

Approximately a half million mental patients are still resident in state mental hospitals on any given day, in addition to those cared for in hospitals administered by the Veterans Administration. What of them, in relation to the community? Although voluntary admissions are increasing, the great majority of patients in state mental hospitals are committed to the hospital by court order and must remain there until the medical staff decides that they may either be released on leave or discharged.

In the past, because of public fear of mental illness, state mental hospitals were usually constructed in isolated, rural settings. Physicians and other personnel were employed by the state, standards of treatment were established by the state health or mental health authority, and the hospital operated as a separate and closed institution. This is still true to a large extent. Mental hospital standards are extremely uneven from state to state. In most of them, once a patient enters the hospital admitting ward, his personal physician can have no further part in his treatment. In addition, although some of the most brilliant and dedicated physicians have practiced and are practicing in the state mental hospital system, it is undeniably true that some physicians who cannot meet required standards to be licensed to practice medicine in a community, can practice in mental hospitals. This is not necessarily because the physician is inadequately qualified from a professional standpoint; often there are restrictions of residence or other matters not related to medical competence. No matter what the reason, the situation has created a chasm between physicians in the community and physicians in the mental hospital. Fortunately, this too is changing.

A Mental Hospital Improvement Program, supported by federal funds, has enabled hospitals for the mentally ill and institutions for the mentally retarded to establish pilot, demonstration projects that are helping to bring the hospital program closer to the regional community in a variety of ways. Through liaison between a mental hospital and a college or university, student nurses, social workers, teachers of mentally retarded children, and others receive a portion of their training in classes provided by the mental hospital staff. Volunteers from the community are being put to effective use in therapeutic programs designed to prepare the mental patient to return to life in his community. Mental hospitals are increasing rehabilitative services, occupational training, and job-finding programs for patients who no longer need to be hospitalized. The role of the mental hospital, therefore, is changing, but it is still organized and operated as a separate system.

In looking toward the future, when most mental patients will be treated within the community, the question arises as to the fate of today's mental hospital as we now know it. Until more knowledge comes from research and continuing treatment progress, some psychiatric patients will continue to need hospitalization for periods beyond the ability of the general hospital psychiatric service to supply. The mental hospital will undoubtedly continue to be the place in which the chronically and severely mentally ill will be treated. But, in addition, other explorations are under way. In recent years, physicians have found that many mental patients, especially the elderly, although sent to mental hospitals for treatment because of overt bizarre behavior, are in actuality suffering from physical illness that should receive appropriate medical or surgical treatment. Malnutrition, vitamin deficiencies, and cardiac conditions can be corrected; when they are, in many instances, the psychiatric disorder disappears. Too often the patient remains in the mental hospital because there is no appropriate nursing home or other facility for the chronically ill patient within his community. Some mental hospital patient populations today are made up in the majority of persons over 65 years of age.

Leaders in mental hospital administration, facing this reality, are experimenting with treatment environments inside the mental hosptal to provide care for the chronically ill and elderly person who is not primarily suffering emotional disturbance. Open wards, community visiting, and recreational programs are increasing in the enlightened mental hospitals. Their success causes some health professionals to hope that these facilities will be used to a large extent in the future to treat chronic illnesses of any kind requiring hospitalization and to serve as research centers for chronic illness in general and the severe psychiatric disorders in particular. Such plans are now being debated, because the professional at work in the mental hospital system, like any other established health facility, has resisted change, fearing that autonomy and sovereignty were threatened. There is increased need and opportunity to strengthen relationships among mental hospitals, community mental health centers, and all the other community health facilities. New construction for mental hospitals should be considered in the same terms of regional planning recommended for general hospital construction and should also be approved solely on the basis of need in the area under consideration.

The Moving Facility

Since more people in the United States live in cities today than in rural areas, the concerns of the urban medical facilities bulk larger. However, no matter how our cities rot in the center, sprawl into suburbs, and hold millions of persons in thrall, the country is still made up of plains and hills and mountains and canyons that are even today the wide open spaces in which many of us live and in which the residents must be provided with health services. Sometimes, it requires a flying ambulance to provide continuity of care. In at least one state, a flying psychiatrist gives supervision to clinics throughout the state. In parts of Appalachia, hospitals are establishing satellite facilities in out-of-the-way localities, and from those satellites treatment teams go into the hills and the hollows periodically to give service to residents of extremely isolated and small communities. There is no lack of innovation in providing rural health services, but there is a lack of efficient organization among local communities which must now plan for joint regional operations to serve their residents. The Hill-Burton hospital construction program has been effective in providing needed construction funds on a weighted basis to areas with low per-capita incomes, making it possible for them to match funds at a lower proportion. Hospital construction in such areas has attracted health personnel, has stimulated young residents of the area to enter the health professions as a career, and is making possible the use of additional indigenous personnel as health aides and other vocational occupations. It will next be necessary to adapt rural health care to the resources potentially available within the area, and to import, on a regular basis, the specialized personnel necessary to provide health services.

Fragmentation and Duplication

Although the community objective must be correlation of services, this does not rule out service duplication when that duplication brings better care at reasonable rates to the community. In urban areas composed of hundreds of thousands and millions of individuals, it is obvious that many hospitals are needed and that each of them will include services provided by some of the others. The essential considerations are coordination of effort, evaluation of need for those services and facilities which are duplicated, and assurance that quality is maintained. This is as it should be. However, services that can best be provided jointly must be integrated.

The hospital of tomorrow, as the facility in which the greatest numbers of skilled personal health personnel are assembled, must also work in concert with others to make sure the supply of that personnel is adequate. Educational institutions — graduate and undergraduate professional schools, junior colleges, and technical schools — engaged in the education of health personnel, have the responsibility to provide patient-oriented training for every member of the health team; hospitals can play an increasing role in these endeavors. If this occurs, it will undoubtedly follow that clinical research will spread among a larger number of institutions, rather than being confined primarily to today's teaching hospitals. This too will affect the size of the hospitals and their location. The modern physician, trained in an environment that included research facilities, searches for a hospital affiliation that will permit him to continue clinical research. And, with effective administration, the interplay of all these factors should allow the hospital to maintain independence of policy, while adhering to mutually beneficial standards and areas of joint provision of the services that every community seeks to provide.

CHAPTER VII

Organization and Management of Resources

In the United States, one of the stereotypes of the twentieth century is "the organization man." He has been emulated, ridiculed, and used as the basis for a great deal of satiric and ironic humor. Satiric comment usually occurs when men rebel against something that exists, must exist, but yet does not operate successfully enough to meet with general approval. No one today will argue too strongly against the need for organization and management, but almost everyone will argue about their patterns and operations. This is certainly true within the debate of the methods to achieve and deliver community health services. While it is neither possible nor desirable to develop a single pattern that might be applied to the entire nation, it is feasible to suggest mechanisms which encourage constructive experimentation in practical patterns of organization.

For administrative purposes, the comprehensive and inclusive entity to be organized and managed is a correlated system of community health services, offered by private, public, and voluntary agencies. Because, although interrelated, problems of administration vary, the services should be organized under two categories — comprehensive personal health services and comprehensive environmental health services. The basic resources that must be available in sufficient quantity and quality to meet community need are men, money, and material. Each community, in other words, must have as the tools with which organizers and administrators can work, sufficient resources in manpower, in finance, and in health facilities to serve the population of the

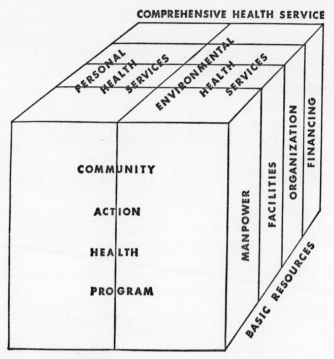

Figure 3. The community health services cube.

community by meeting its demands for personal health services and protection against environmental hazards.

To reach this objective, an essential condition is health administration that clearly defines the roles and responsibilities of the individual, the physician, the community, its agencies, and its civic leadership in putting to maximum, effective use the resources of men, money, and material. It is at this point that consideration of administration, organization, and management ceases to retain the static boundaries of a textbook concept and becomes a dynamic and vivid controversy; for those who must administer a system of community health services are immediately faced with the decisions which will affect every sector of the community. There are conflicting values of administration in planning, fiscal responsibility, supervisory responsibility, and responsibility for provision of services. Manpower must somehow be assembled and supplied, even in the face of shortage of supply, so that it will meet the need for its services. The correlation and financing of health facilities is today entwined in the concepts of regionalism and overlapping communities, as administrators seek a workable confederation for planning facilities on a regional basis, securing and utilizing funds, and coordinating their services for the use of every resident of that regional community.

The health industry must realize that its success, in competition for the tools it needs to do the job, will depend on full use of its brains and its brawn. "Brains and brawn" is the label for the composite of organizational and managerial knowledge — know-how — plus the amount of political muscle necessary to secure public acceptance and support of the organization specifically proposed. The attributes of Florence Nightingale are unchanged, but they are not quite enough in 1966.

New Organizational Patterns

As communities search for an organizational renaissance in providing health services, Commission studies indicate that they do so on the basis of four assumptions, or premises, based on modern community living habits and mobilities. Each individual is now a member of a large number of congruent or overlapping health communities. Since no one individual can relate comfortably to so many, the number of such communities should be reduced. Since no two communities or regions are exactly alike, local and regional needs and differences can best be dealt with by the residents of the community involved, with the help of additional leadership, guidelines, and financial support provided at the state and national level. The principal responsibility for establishing patterns for effective community organization lies with the states, even though it is increasingly shared or strongly affected by actions of the federal government. Planning and administration of health facilities is intimately and inextricably involved with the planning and administration of health services.

In discussing new organizational patterns for health services, the Commission arrived at the opinion that the state is the jurisdictional entity on which attention must be primarily focused. For, despite the continuing demand for independence among smaller, local communities, and despite a greatly increased participation by the federal government in matters pertaining to health and welfare, the state still holds the mandate stated in the Constitution of the United States as the governmental center of all power not specifically held by the federal government. In like measure, all counties, townships, and cities are political creatures of the state and their powers have been delegated to them by the state. Therefore, while there is a definite tendency to develop regional approaches (interstate and intrastate) to health services, by planning for them on the basis of geographical areas whose residents wish to secure common community objectives, it still seems feasible to consider the state as the filter, the arbiter, and in many instances, the level at which plans and programs are initiated. In this context, the Commission considers the state as an administrative level for both governmental and voluntary agencies.

A typical problem facing organizers of community health service programs, governmental and voluntary, is the decision as to the size of jurisdictions for local services and the relative advantages and disadvantages of state administrative districts, as compared with districts composed of one or more existing units. Local health agencies wish to take a prominent part in the administration of health care; if this is to be an effective pattern, modification and change in the boundaries of local health jurisdictions must be made, in most, if not all, the states. Governmental health agencies, for the most part, have been established to dovetail with political boundaries, and, consequently, health jurisdictions usually conform to them also. Voluntary agencies, which in the past tended to use these same boundaries, are increasingly moving away from them.

There is now general agreement that many of these areas are too limited in population, and therefore in funding potential, to provide either efficient administration or adequate financing of such an expensive program as health care. In addition, even though the form, if not the reality, of administration and financing has been limited by governmental jurisdictional boundaries, physicians, hospitals, and voluntary agencies have not drawn their clientele from the area bounded by existing local subdivisions. Health and welfare associations and voluntary health agencies have already consolidated units in and around metropolitan areas, and public health officers are rapidly arriving at the belief that public health jurisdictions must be reshaped to follow the natural lines of community trade areas.

Political considerations raise problems not specific to health affairs, but crucial as the setting for health action. The most significant political issue in community health organization is that of the revision of outmoded, overlapping, and ambiguous jurisdictions. Health service administrative areas must be efficiently functional in terms of major health problems. Some of these problems can and should be handled within the area of the political community, but not all health problems can be circumscribed by traditional community, state, and national boundaries.

The planning, organization, and delivery of community health services must be based on the concept of a "community of solution" — that is, environmental health problem-sheds and health marketing areas, rather than primarily on political jurisdictions. [A]

Where the community of solution of a health problem requires coordinated action by several jurisdictions, appropriate use should be made of compacts, agreements, and interstate authorities, as well as other innovative procedures for expediting delivery of health services. [A-5] There are currently in existence several procedures which allow for grouping among the traditional jurisdictional areas. There have been many consolidations of county health departments, both with other counties and with city departments. Interstate and intrastate compacts are being explored and expanded in an effort to give some elasticity to political jurisdictions whose funding is currently limited by the tax levy agreed to by residents. Their health programs also are limited by the wishes of the citizens who adopt or reject health legislative proposals and who place in office those executives and legislators who, they think, will hold taxes to reasonable limits while sponsoring measures designed to provide good health services. The existence of metropolitan units or authorities — sometimes crossing state boundaries — to administer planning for water, sewage, parks, tunnels, airports, and pollution control indicates some willingness to take a more sophisticated view

of necessity by superseding the authority of local political jurisdictions, but opponents of such procedures continue to speak as
vehemently from their viewpoint as do the proponents.

Organization for community health services must be directly
related to planning for those services. The experiences of the
Commission's community studies (in Chattanooga and Reno, for
example, as noted in Chapter I) validate the concept that the
planning, organization, and delivery of community health services must be on a community of solution basis. To provide the
wide perspective that such planning requires for the entire state,
each state should have a State Health Policy and Planning Commission, responsible to the governor, to advise him on health
planning for the state. Such a commission would be representative of governmental, private, and voluntary groups. It would
have no administrative functions but would, by the plans it made,
set the framework for administration of health services in the
state whether these services were offered by governmental, private, or voluntary groups.*

A major function of this commission would be to examine,
with the state health department, the state's pattern of health
jurisdictions and recommend groupings of one or more political
units as problem-sheds for environmental health services or as
health marketing areas for personal health services. [A-1] These
groupings should correspond to the geographic regions from
which communities can draw every needed support. Each region
should have available an adequate supply of every health skill
and resource. In addition, regions established for personal health
services should have a fully equipped and staffed medical center.

Both providers and consumers of health care should participate
in the development of regional plans, and every community or
rural area should be included in one region or another. Reasonable attention should be given to the established trend of patterns for health care, as well as to traditional political boundaries of cities, counties, and states. Boundaries of the regions
established should be regularly reassessed and revised so that

---

* That the Commission's concern in this matter was shared in other quarters was
evidenced by the introduction of federal legislation on this subject during the
drafting of this report.

they can be continuously adapted to the changing dimensions of health problems.

These regions should be established as organized units for the administration of health services. [A-2] Voluntary and private agencies would determine whether they needed to reconstitute their own administrative districts or whether to rely on cooperation and communication between local units. The function of the State Health Policy and Planning Commission would be to stimulate and promote the regionalization needed for efficient delivery of both environmental and personal health services, no matter who supplies them. Every region should have a health planning council, organized on a permanent basis, under top-echelon citizen and professional leadership, financed from a variety of sources, responsible for general health services and facilities planning within the context of the region's total spectrum of health services, and coordinated with the planning of other community, regional, and state planning agencies, especially the State Health Policy and Planning Commission. [A-3]

Although such regional planning groups should be established as soon as possible, regions and communities can take appropriate interim measures which will help pave the way for the planning councils. One step would be the encouragement of cooperative interagency planning — governmental and voluntary — of service programs and facilities, in such manner as to assure joint utilization of those services and facilities. [A-4]

It must be recognized that the necessary resources — men, money, and material — stem from efforts of the private and public sectors of each community. Although it has in many ways been an uneasy partnership, the joint activity of public and private leadership in health services has developed significantly in recent years. That development must be accelerated in the foreseeable future if the correlation of community health services is to be obtained by adapting our present modes of operation, rather than changing them entirely.

Another trend which must be further developed across the country in the immediate future is the organizational unity of community health and community hospital responsibilities. To achieve this, there must be a closer working relationship between health departments and the departments which administer publicly financed hospitals. Lack of this sort of administrative coordination is one of the major causes of piecemeal health care for the medically indigent, for, when many individuals and agencies are responsible for the management of a patient, often no one accepts total responsibility. With the establishment of coordinating administrative bodies, communities can more easily identify health problems and move effectively to solve them. The failures in providing adequate health care in health facilities are usually not the failures of individual persons, but failures of the system — lack of communication, continuity, follow-up, or the fixing of responsibility. A recent review of a 400-bed municipal hospital in New York City, for example, brought to light the fact that the shortage of nurses was so acute that patient care had arrived at a critical level. This situation exists across the country in many disciplines besides nursing, and it will be intensified as people take advantage of Medicare benefits unless coordination of staffing, among other things, is improved.

The New York City Interdepartmental Health Council's activities are illustrative of methods by which the delivery of health care can be significantly improved. New York City aligned the municipal hospitals with strong voluntary teaching hospitals and medical schools; the result was a great improvement in medical staffing that made it possible for each institution to maintain its accreditation. This was achieved through an affiliation contract arrangement, which has been extended to cover nursing services, as a pilot project in one municipal hospital. Working through the Interdepartmental Health Council, it has been possible to set standards that apply to all medical institutions providing care for needy patients for whom the city has assumed responsibility. It is conceivable that this kind of administrative organization could be used for further experimental, pilot projects in a community, in which, for example, adequate personnel and adequate standards could be provided for organized home care programs. In addition, by demonstrating the value of coordinated planning and administration among publicly financed health agencies, including hospitals, public health and hospital departments will be providing a model that can be adapted to the administrative needs of privately financed health facilities, again including hospitals.

This kind of coordinated administration is needed not only in cities, but also in states. A problem common to all states has been that of differing ways of handling publicly financed health care. States have not only different definitions of "residence" but also different regulations about eligibility, usually based on that residence. The family which moves from one state to another while the mother is pregnant is seldom able to get publicly financed care in the new state, even though the family was eligible for and had been receiving such care in the original state. Similarly, the child or other family member taken ill in the new state is not covered. After 1969, no state participating in Title XIX public assistance programs ("Grants to States for Medical Assistance Programs," of the *Social Security Amendments of 1965*) can deny medical aid on the basis that the applicant has not lived in the state long enough. However, each participating state will continue to contribute part of the cost of Title XIX programs, and, if a state does not have a strong program, or elects not to participate, the problem is still with us — or more precisely still with the person needing care. Some state welfare programs will be unaffected by Title XIX. Other aid programs should seek similar ways to make sure that by moving his family with him to seek employment in a new city, a man does not jeopardize his family's eligibility for needed health care.

Still largely unrecognized, except by the immediate communities involved, are the community health services problems caused or compounded by large concentrations of federal services such as military installations. These are not, primarily, health care problems, as most such installations have their own military hospitals or clinics. But such concentrations of manpower bring with them community problems of restaurant sanitation, sewage disposal, water supply, and venereal disease that the local community is ill-equipped to handle without additional resources. Some program similar to that worked out for schools needs to be undertaken for health services.

Tooling Up for Health Services: Modern Management

To a large extent, the ultimate success of any change in organizational patterns will rest on the quality of management of each part of the comprehensive community health services program. It is in the area of management that most health professionals are far less skilled than they are in professional and technical matters. Many agencies and institutions continue to use outdated organization and management procedures at a time when modern, sophisticated procedures are available to them. It will not be possible to meet the impact of public demand for health services in the immediate future unless modern management establishes the routine utilization of the best techniques available. How, for example, is it possible even to think of providing continuity of care for a patient unless that patient's records are assembled, stored for referral, and transmitted from one health care facility to another, as required by his treatment needs? In protecting the confidentialness of patients' records, the health industry has perhaps created an even larger problem; for, when one agency retains the records, the next agency must begin all over again and, as many a weary patient has discovered, the same questions are asked and answered time after time, diagnoses are arrived at again and again — only to result in another referral rather than effective treatment.

Similar remodeling must occur in methods of providing all the managerial services necessary to the efficient operation of a health program. It may seem elemental to state in a report such as this that the principal services provided by management are legal counsel, fiscal services, personnel, planning, statistical and office services, and records and report systems. But, in many a rural area in this nation, such services, routine in many cities, exist in very inadequate forms or do not exist at all. Health agency functions frequently have legal or quasi-legal aspects which require legal services. These include the preparation of codes, administrative rules, licensing, drafting, legislation, contract negotiations, the conduct of hearings, and the issuance of orders. Fiscal services are necessary to consolidate various agency expenses into a comprehensive agency budget. They are also necessary in relations with state budget officials, in applying for and administering federal grants and other funds, and in the disbursement of funds, preparation of financial reports, and maintenance of financial records.

No community health service program can exist without effective personnel services — not only a service within the individual agency, but a personnel service designed to meet the manpower needs of the entire, specific health trade area. The recruitment, training, and placement of able personnel are the primary responsibilities of the personnel service. Another basic function is a liaison with the relevant civil service or merit systems in operation in the area, as well as with labor and management bargaining groups whose decisions establish rates of pay and other working conditions for health personnel. The personnel service, in addition to providing information on such standards, should also serve in an advisory capacity while standards are under negotiation.

The implementation of new programs, whether by legislative mandate or on the agency's own initiative, requires the services of people expert in applied organizational theory and the development of systems and procedures. The continuing evaluation and improvement of current programs can also be advanced by the use of administrative planning personnel. Most areas, even the smallest and most remote communities, keep some kind of health statistical records, but the paucity of comprehensive health data on a national basis shows the nationwide need to develop an automated system of data collection, storage, and retrieval, not only on statistics of births, deaths, marriages, and reportable diseases, but in a far wider area pertaining to all facets of health and disease. Such information will provide the raw materials for the research projects so necessary in improving personal and environmental health services. Additionally, automatic data processing makes statistical data more valuable in measuring the effectiveness of programs and in testing alternate models of action.

We have become accustomed to the use of automated techniques of program analysis, research, and operation in the armed forces, the space program, and other sectors of both the public and private industrial world. But we have been extremely slow to adapt similar tools for use in providing health services. Many of these techniques are being used, but in most instances, the coordinated use is limited to a relatively few major medical centers, and even these have not as yet put them to maximum use. The health industry task in this field is to spread the knowledge of modern organizational structures and management processes and to establish regional centers and information clearinghouses whose knowledge can be made available not only to large medical centers but to small hospitals or direct service health plans and the individual physician in rural areas.

It is evident that, if each local community health program includes the administrative organization and management services mentioned here, it will become far simpler to negotiate and administer interstate, intercounty, and intercity contracts and other agreements for sharing the operation and financing of joint health services. Effective administration will also enable community health programs to take advantage of the variety of funding aids available from official and voluntary agencies which can help to finance the cost of health services.

A new concept for the organization of health services has been evolved, affecting both official and voluntary agencies. New partnerships, differing for different problems and differing communities of solution, can more effectively solve health problems. State-local, federal-state, federal-region, and state-intrastate regions are now being established for this purpose; newer combinations will be developed as more experience is gained. For administering health activities, in addition to federal and state health agencies, we can develop within the nation regional health jurisdictions that encompass the community of solution for personal or environmental health problems. Within the states, we can develop intrastate regions along similar lines to cover every community, rural or urban. These four jurisdictions can operate effectively side by side if they are planned and administered wisely and adapted to changes as they occur.

Partners in Progress:
The Governments

The principle of joint action through local, state, and national authorities is inherent in the system of federal government. The delivery of comprehensive community health services requires the full implementation of that principle and exploration of its full potential in a partnership of governmental and voluntary institutions. Legislation has recognized this partnership. Major health legislation commits the federal partner to support research by competent investigators and to help finance a significant portion of environmental and personal health services; it challenges the other partners to fulfill their roles in meeting the nation's pressing needs in this field.

The template is yet to be cut for the broadened dimensions of this partnership for health. Meanwhile, officials at all levels of government and individuals in many voluntary services are seeking to design the organizational and funding patterns with which the health partners can jointly provide and deliver a constellation of services of superior quality. The creation of new designs for health responsive to the needs inherent in phenomenal growth and change demands constant reexamination and restructuring of resources, roles, relationships, institutions, and instruments on the part of all governments and on the part of the private sector as well.

The tone of this nationwide effort is conveyed in the words of John W. Gardner, Secretary of the United States Department of Health, Education, and Welfare, in an address to the American Medical Association, October 1, 1965: "I believe that the federal government and various sectors of the private world — whether they are corporations or universities or professions — can enter into fruitful collaboration. I am convinced this collaboration can take a form that guarantees the continued integrity of private groups, that preserves local initiative, and that maintains the pluralism and public-private balance that we all treasure."

The States: Authority and Responsibility

Throughout this report, the Commission has reiterated awareness of the changes that must be made to adapt local health jurisdictions to population shifts and to changes in the nature of the health problems, so that health services will be available where they are needed — as the primary criterion — even if new patterns of cooperation must be established to achieve this end. Many variants of governmental collaboration will be developed in the next few years, based on the traditions, customs, and funding patterns of each community, in relation to those of neighboring geographical areas sharing congruent service problems. However, the governmental unit which should maintain and exercise the major public authority for provision of health services within its jurisdiction is the state. The state not only has this basic constitutional authority, but also, as a political and territorial unit, has both a broader jurisdiction and a greater fiscal capacity than any single local community. Given the dimensions of the health needs of our society today, it is imperative that state capacities for service be strengthened so that they will be better able to deal with those aspects of comprehensive health in which they have a special responsibility and to support and facilitate the strengthening of local jurisdictions.

Every state should have a single, strong, well-financed, professionally staffed, official health agency with sufficient authority and funds to carry out its responsibilities. The state should assure every community of coverage by an official health agency and access to the complete range of community health services.

This state agency must be able to work effectively with federal agencies, to provide all the environmental and personal health services for which it is responsible, to stimulate and support the development of local health units that will provide official health

agency services to local communities, to take leadership in broad-
ening the scope and quality of health services available to its
communities, and to respond positively to the health needs of
the public.

This single agency, in which all the major health programs of
the state government should be concentrated, would be able to
coordinate the various environmental, preventive, curative, and
rehabilitative components into a comprehensive health service
system. It should be responsible for setting the health standards
of other state programs even though they may be a secondary
activity of another agency. [L]

Health programs have become a crazy quilt of disconnected
and rambling services. Related services have been divorced from
each other: the preventive from the therapeutic; the medical
from the sanitary; and the rehabilitative from both the preventive
and the therapeutic. The coordination of agency health services,
by the very magnitude and complexity of the agencies involved,
has become, like the weather, something to talk about but about
which people believe little can be done. The consumer may
easily become confused and chagrined when looking for help.
Lack of coordination increases the cost of services significantly
and aggravates an already acute manpower shortage.

Public welfare departments, for example, have become increasingly involved in the administration of health services as a
segment of their responsibility for individuals on public assistance. Consequently, closer integration between health and
welfare agencies is imperative, with the immediate objective of
effective coordination of their health activities.

The fact that state mental hygiene departments have developed
as agencies separate from health departments has resulted in
divided responsibility in the health field. This is inconsistent with
the evolution of the concept of mental health programming with
a locus in the state hospital to emerging concepts of community
based preventive and treatment services. This fragmentation
could be corrected through the consolidation of all state health
activities in a strong state health agency.

States should take steps to effect the consolidation of all their
official health services (including mental health, school health,

mental retardation, the administration of medical care programs for the indigent, and the medical aspects of rehabilitation) in a single agency. [L-1] The state should assign to this health agency responsibility for developing and/or maintaining all programs necessary to protect people from environmental hazards and from poor quality health services, and that it be specifically charged to initiate action to meet new and changing health needs. [L-2] A strong state health agency would thus be the principal governmental device to put into effect the determinations made by the State Health Policy and Planning Commission described in Chapter VII.

The existing official health agencies in the 50 states exhibit marked variations in structure, functions, programs, and personnel. If the leadership role recommended for these agencies is to be exercised in each state it will require a well-organized professional staff commensurate with the broadened functions and responsibilities. As a primary requisite, each state health department must have adequate funds and enforcement authority, and the state must secure for it sufficient financial support provided in the most flexible manner possible, with proper safeguards. [L-3]

Local Health Departments

Local health departments also vary in quality from state to state and from town to town, and the exercise of leadership in broadening the scope and quality of health services available to communities would be a key role of a strong state health agency. In carrying out this role, each state should stimulate and support the development of local health units in such a manner that every community within its jurisdiction would be effectively served by an official health agency and would have access to appropriate health services, official or otherwise.

A "local" health department may be responsible for service to a city, a county, a city and county community, or several counties combined in a region, depending on the configuration which can best carry out the duties jointly determined by state and local authorities. Local community leaders should be encouraged to begin thinking in terms of clusters of cities, towns, and related rural areas which make natural, or at least organizationally feasible and defensible, regions for improving the health of the area. A local health department's responsibilities, duties, structure, staff, and relationships have been well described in the 1964 policy statement of the American Public Health Association.*

Local health agencies are most effective when they anticipate and respond to the needs of the community. Therefore, the local health department should be expected to assume the leadership in planning comprehensive health services and organizing those services which it can best establish and deliver; it should be so financed and staffed with full-time personnel especially trained in the public health sciences that it can do so. Such planning should have top priority. [L-4]

To preserve appropriate local autonomy in health matters and to build citizen interest in their own health problems and plans, the state should delegate as many of its functions to the local health unit as can be properly and effectively carried out within the community concerned. [L-5] It is also appropriate, where local health units do not exist, that the state health agency inform the citizens of the reasons why the local health department must be organized, and establish the amount of support that each community can expect to receive from the state health agency.

Financial support is a primary requirement for successful local operation. Local governments depend heavily on limited tax resources; their sources of tax revenue are smaller by far than those of the state and federal governments. Therefore, they must depend in varying degrees on state and federal funds to augment local health programs. The means by which the state and the federal government can best share the financial load of the nation's health activities is increasingly under review. More funds for local health services will be required if comprehensive programs are developed, and certain principles are important guides in the provision of these funds. Local governments are dependent on the state for their power and responsibilities; therefore, the

* "The Local Health Department — Services and Responsibilities." A policy statement adopted by the Governing Council of the American Public Health Association, November 10, 1963. *American Journal of Public Health,* January 1964, pp. 131-139. Available in reprint form from APHA, 1790 Broadway, New York, 10019.

state has an obligation to see that local units are adequately financed. Increased state aid should contain financial incentives for any necessary reform in structure and organization of local health agencies, including appropriate consolidations. The federal government should assist in financing community health services through the states by awarding grants in as flexible a manner as possible, consistent with the maintenance of standards of quality. Categorical project grants should be employed only to assist in solving specific serious health problems currently needing special emphasis; categorical formula grants should be reviewed periodically as to accomplishments and phased into the basic grant when the categorical approach is no longer justified; and the basic (general) formula health grant should be increased both absolutely and as a proportion of total grants. [L-6]

The Federal Government: The Import of Federal Legislation for Community Health Services

The strength of the wind of change is dramatized by the widespread implications of that which is enacted into law. The word is no longer "if" or "when," but "how"? In search of attitudes toward the way in which legislation will affect community health services, the Commission has concentrated on the possible effects of certain federal programs on health and on the personnel who will provide the services.

Heart, Cancer, and Stroke. Medical schools, hospitals, and other health facilities will be assisted in establishing and operating regionally coordinated medical programs for heart disease, cancer, stroke, and associated ills. As these developments provide for regional geographic grouping of research and treatment programs, they will affect health practice far beyond the three diseases on which they are primarily focused. While this attack is aimed at three major causes of death, it is also a national effort to establish community health services for three important causes of disability, and will probably result in an improvement in many health services. Medical schools, research facilities, private physicians, local hospitals, and public and voluntary health agencies in given regions will be working together in a regional integration of facilities and services that may well be extended to other areas. Training of physicians, nurses, medical social workers, and the allied health groups should be favorably influenced. The possibility of better treatment for children, as well as for older patients, will be involved.

As is true for any vital new effort, problems of administration will arise. As they are solved, the solutions may be adaptable for other health needs. For example, the requirement that patients treated in regional centers be referred by their physician focuses attention on the need for individuals to have personal physicians. Record systems using electronic data processing which may be useful to other health programs will likely be developed. It is of interest that among the criteria for judging applications for development of a heart, cancer, and stroke program is the extent to which all the health resources of the region have been taken into consideration in the planning and/or establishment of the program. This is essentially the requirement that the Commission made in establishing criteria for the 21 community self-studies conducted under its auspices.

By requiring collaboration on a national scale, the heart, cancer, and stroke program opens a door to new methods and new combinations of facilities in the treatment of illness. Many of the recommendations of the Commission, which have been made separately in this report, can be put into action under the act, as an instrument for development of health services on a regional basis.

Medical Care of the Aged. Under the 1965 Amendments to the Social Security Act, nearly all persons over 65 years of age are covered by a basic plan that provides payment for most hospital and nursing home costs, excepting physicians' fees, through Social Security taxes paid by employers and employees. A voluntary supplementary insurance plan covers most physicians' charges and costs of certain other medical services not paid under the basic plans. The voluntary plan is financed by monthly payments by each enrollee, matched by payments from the federal government. In addition, medical assistance for medically indigent aged, blind, and disabled persons and for dependent children and their parents is provided by law. Health service leaders must find ways to manage health services so that the increase of requests for medical care under the insurance plan will not impair the quality of the care available.

Major innovations of these programs, with important implications for future health care demands, are the extension of the social insurance mechanism as a means of paying for medical care for those over 65, and the inclusion of psychiatric care in insured benefits. For the first time, the federal government will match state money payments for individuals on public assistance who are in mental hospitals. The federal government will also share the costs of medical care of the medically indigent in mental hospitals, if the state elects to provide such medical assistance, even though such persons are not receiving public assistance. These provisions will result in more adequate financing of treatment for the mentally ill, and a more equitable sharing of the cost of care between the state and federal governments.

To every person concerned with community health services, these massive new programs pose a challenge. They must be put into operation in a manner that reinforces and strengthens comprehensiveness and integration of community health services. Depending on our ingenuity, or lack of it, these programs will be either strong forces for better health care or they will be disruptive.

Other Programs Related to Community Health Services

Rehabilitation. Flexibility in financing and administering state rehabilitation programs and expansion and improvement of those programs, particularly for the mentally retarded and other groups presenting special vocational rehabilitative problems, can result from federal legislation. At the same time, grants for the construction and initial staffing of rehabilitation facilities and sheltered workshops will continue to help communities deal with such problems.

Mental Illness and Retardation. Legislation has focused attention on the needs of the mentally retarded and mentally ill for services in specialized settings, and on community needs for financial assistance in making those services available, including facilities and staff. The needs for training of personnel and research have also been highlighted. It is the Commission's position that such facilities, as they are constructed and placed in operation throughout the country, should be integral parts of the total comprehensive community health service system.

Immunization. Community health planning is affected by such federal programs as those assisting state and local health departments to expand mass immunization programs against polio, diphtheria, whooping cough, tetanus, and measles.

General and Special Health Services. Aid to states and communities for general and special health services, including grants for migratory workers, the chronically ill, and the aged and grants for research to improve special services, extends a community's capacity to cope with the needs.

Education and Research. Legislation has influenced developments in other areas of benefit to all elements of the community health system, such as services, facilities, training, and research related to medical libraries; health research facilities; and education of the health professions, including not only financial aid for the construction of schools of medicine, dentistry, osteopathy, and optometry but also new and expanded programs of scholarships and loan assistance.

Poverty. Health services are affected by federal programs to counteract poverty and the acute problems associated with it, and the Commission urges that health departments and the Office of Economic Opportunity cooperate in bringing the available resources to bear on health related problems.

Water Pollution. Federal water pollution control programs can establish quality standards for interstate streams in those states which fail to take action establishing acceptable standards. Grant funds for the construction of waste treatment works have been increased, both for individual pollution control projects and for projects which will be helpful to several adjacent communities.

Water Resources. The threat to water supply posed by increased usage for industrial and agricultural purposes is of concern to the federal government. Basic legislation provides for federal grants each year over a ten-year period in matching funds to states for planning water projects, and establishes a cabinet-level Water Resources Council to coordinate the creation of river basin commissions for regional water resources planning. To improve the quantity and quality of rural water supplies, grants and increased loans for water facilities in rural agricultural areas are included.

Air Pollution. Legislation related to clean air establishes a mechanism to require control of emissions from gasoline and diesel engines and sets standards. The Secretary of the United States Department of Health, Education, and Welfare is authorized to construct, staff, and equip whatever facilities are necessary to carry out controls. The legislation also launches a new program of grants for research to improve methods of collecting, handling, and disposing of solid wastes.

Drugs. Strengthened controls over hazardous drugs are established to combat illegal traffic in them, reinforce community programs to prevent abuse, and counteract a growing threat to health.

Every community has a responsibility to share in implementing these broad programs. The challenge will be to correlate the administration of these promising governmental endeavors to achieve their intent, to reduce fragmented and wasteful procedures, and thereby to serve the public. The size and nature of the programs will require extremely skillful administration, a flexible approach in their implementation, extension of facilities for treatment and research, and the training of large numbers of additional professional and administrative personnel.

Federal Grants for Public Health

The keys to much of the success with which the challenge of correlation will be met are in the hands of the official public health agency — federal, regional, state, or local.

Federal grants-in-aid have proven a very effective method for providing assistance to bring some underdeveloped health activities up to national standards and to aid communities in maintaining their facilities at satisfactory levels. Grants should also be available to stimulate communities to provide new services as needed. The federal grant system is enormous and complex, however, and should be reviewed periodically in order to assure value received in the distribution and utilization of public funds for health.

Among the conditions which should be changed is the usual time lag between the authorization of grant funds and the appropriation of those funds. Since grants are made for specific time periods, the time lag in a one-year grant, for example, may mean that anywhere from two to four months of that period are lost, if funds are not appropriated for the entire twelve-month period and no carry-over provisions are included.

Further, categorical grants have increased in proportion to general grants. Because the categorical funds are available for narrow projects and are rigidly controlled, a state or local health department is often unable to make the best use of them and in some instances may be unable to use them at all. At the same time, the same health department may be unable to secure enough funds to maintain its general, ongoing, basic health program.

There is an immediate need for a consistent policy to shape the federal grants-in-aid system. Such a policy should delineate the health responsibilities for each of the levels of government — federal, state, and local — and should support basic state and local planning and health services, provide special grants to stimulate new health programs, and require achievement of objectives in accordance with sound administrative practices.

The adoption of legislation designed to achieve the fullest cooperation and coordination of activities among levels of government is essential in order to improve their operation, to improve the administration of grants-in-aid to the states, and to provide for periodic congressional review of federal grants-in-aid.

Federal Grants for Research in Public Health Departments

The provision of additional research funds for specific public health needs, such as air and water pollution control and solid waste disposal, will of course benefit all interests. Such specific projects are vital and project research should be a continuing activity of all public health departments, related to conditions that develop and needs that can be predicted and estimated. In addition, since comparatively few official health departments are provided with adequate general research funds through their local and state funding agencies, general support funds for research should be made available by the federal government. These funds should be provided with the intent of furthering the advance of the total research capacity of the health department, including the employment of competent research personnel. [L-7]

To secure such a grant program, the Commission joins with The American Public Health Association and the Association of State and Territorial Health Officers in requesting the Secretary of the Department of Health, Education, and Welfare to inform the directors of fund-granting units under his jurisdiction of the necessity for examining their policies and procedures with a particular view to making available General Research Support funds to develop and strengthen the research potential of official health departments. The present eligibility rules for such General Research Support grants through the National Institutes of Health should be changed so that funds for health research received from any unit of the Department of Health, Education, and Welfare may be counted in establishing eligibility.

Since criticism of the performance of health departments often centers on their lack of initiative in seeking solutions for new and complex problems, it seems obvious that improvement of staff abilities to enter into and continue basic and applied research is a high priority need, if health department personnel are to assume their share of leadership in improving community health services.

It has been demonstrated that research creates an environment attractive to men of ideas and imagination. Official health agencies will be better able to compete for the talented personnel they need to do the job required of them if they can provide additional research opportunities within their conventional functions, especially in the realm of community planning, health administration, including hospital management, and behavioral factors affecting health.

Coordination of Governmental Health Programs

The establishment by the federal government of an effective mechanism for coordinating and directing its health program in a manner that will strengthen the effectiveness of state and local planning units and health agencies is greatly needed if its full promise is to be realized. The Department of Health, Education, and Welfare may be expected to develop such a mechanism. Federal government health programs and the state and local programs to which they relate will benefit from the singleness of focus of responsibility, organization, information, and direction that should result from better coordination.

Without such coordination, federal agencies tend to be unintentionally disruptive of state and local agencies. The complexity of relationships may be illustrated by listing a number of the units in the Department of Health, Education, and Welfare which administer programs which strongly affect community health administration as well as planning: Public Health Service, Office of Education, Food and Drug Administration, Vocational Rehabilitation Administration, Welfare Administration, and Water Pollution Control Administration. In the Public Health Service alone there are programs for hospitals, environmental engineering, food protection, dental public health, radiation, water supply, chronic diseases, air pollution, accident prevention, immunization, and all manner of health research. Other government agencies that administer relevant health programs include the departments of Labor, Agriculture, Defense, Interior, and Housing and Urban Development as well as the Office of Economic Opportunity, Atomic Energy Commission, Veterans Administration, Selective Service System, and Small Business Administration.

In working to resolve its internal complexities, the federal government has asked for consultation with spokesmen from both private and public health units. Practitioners, hospitals, medical schools, and local agencies share responsibility for working as individuals and as groups in such a manner that the federal funding and service umbrella adds growth without implying subordination, strengthens the partnership without lessening desirable autonomy, and assures accountability without crippling initiative.

This process can succeed only in proportion to the measure of good faith and trust that the partners afford one another in creating a new national health program based on local community organization and operation. In this context, as each government unit moves to define its prerogatives and its limits of activity, so must private institutions, facilities, and agencies accept the public demand for a working health partnership. Each must place the public good above his own particular and specific interests, while sustaining the values of independence and integrity. To do so will require new attitudes and original thinking on the part of many persons concerned, but success in doing so will have a bearing on every individual's opportunity for health, and on the strength and health of the nation.

The Officials' Dilemma

Many means are available to add state and federal funds to local budgets, but the procedures for using them are needlessly complicated. In addition, there is this basic question: What share of the "tax pie," at each government taxing level, shall be allocated to the provision of health services? In modern political America, this question is usually decided at the polls. Then, as legislators face the task of stretching the available funds to meet all the requests, the competition becomes one of political muscle and the interplay of community power structures. The health professions have witnessed, as has everyone else, the results of the public demand for health services, as exemplified in national legislation. They, together with voluntary agencies, universities, and the governments, must recognize this mandate for what it is, and go about the business of preparing their hospitals, clinics, teaching facilities, nursing homes, and all the rest to receive and give quality care to all the people who, in search of health, will shortly come knocking at the door.

CHAPTER IX

Partners in Progress:
The Volunteers

One of the unique characteristics of American life — indelibly stamped "Made in the U.S.A." — is the fact that independent, individual citizens seek and accept responsibility for participation in local, state, and national affairs through voluntary leadership and service. That participation can involve the individual in a broad spectrum of activities, ranging from personal effort to organized effort through associations of individuals linked by a common purpose.

When voluntary citizen participation becomes organized, it becomes part of the diverse system of health programs and services of this nation. What is the voluntary health system like? The answer depends in part on what is meant by "voluntary." Frequently the term is used to describe any agency or institution which is nongovernmental. In this context we see a broad and variegated system.

Many kinds of institutions are involved. Some are business concerns — drug manufacturers, hospital supply corporations, and commercial health insurance companies, for example. There are health programs in industry and business as an integrated part of the personnel management function. A small percentage of hospital care, but a large percentage of nursing home care, is rendered in proprietary institutions. There are, in addition, those in the health professions who are in private practice. All these institutions and persons are voluntary in the sense of being nongovernmental.

There also exists a wide variety of institutions known as voluntary, nonprofit organizations, including nonprofit hospitals, non-profit prepayment plans, national voluntary health agencies, and their state and local counterparts. In this group also are purely local health agencies, voluntary groups with significant but secondary health activities (civic, fraternal, and service groups), professional associations (of physicians, nurses, or dentists) at the national, state, and local levels, and associations of health organizations (hospitals, nursing homes, and health councils). These organizations are governed by boards of directors comprising a wide range of community leadership. They are the home, in large part, of the volunteers — the civic-minded citizens from all walks of life who give of themselves without financial recompense.

Because the health needs and programs of the nation are constantly developing and changing, the programs of voluntary health agencies need constant revision. Some national voluntary health agencies, such as those devoted to the control of cancer, heart disease, and tuberculosis, pursue the problems of specific diseases; others are broader in scope. Sometimes they overlap. They raise large amounts of money through appeals to the public. Provision is needed for periodic review of programs and expenditures through a voluntary coordinating and standard-setting group, such as the National Health Council.

Vast amounts of money are funneled through prepayment, insurance plans, and government to voluntary hospitals and physicians rendering care. Are the benefits properly designed? Are the hospitals efficiently organized? Frequently, standards are set and programs evaluated by voluntary groups. For example, the American Medical Association sets standards for medical internships and residencies. The Association of American Medical Colleges is the instrument through which medical schools constantly seek to improve the education of physicians. The American Hospital Association, among its many concerns, is now exploring new administrative practices and effective methods of centralizing statistics and accounts. The Joint Commission on Accreditation of Hospitals has established standards for and accredits hospitals and nursing homes.

Revision is needed constantly because in our fast-moving world these many voluntary strands can become tangled by virtue of being outdated, excessively duplicative, and confusing. In the variety of local leadership in these agencies there is a unique vitality which must be preserved, but one requiring constant vigilance. Duplication may occur not only between two or more voluntary agencies but also between government and voluntary agencies. Some overlap is inevitable, but the relationship in general should be complementary and mutually supportive.

There are exciting possibilities for the partnership between government and voluntary agencies. Each needs the other for the tremendous thrust that will be required to bring the nation's community health services to the levels of quantity and quality that must be reached. While fruitful collaboration and mutually supportive efforts have played a significant part in the development of many community services, unfortunately, at times the discourse between government and voluntary agencies has been discordant.

The time has come when it should be recognized that the voluntary system has helped to attract a substantial amount of the gross national product to health programs and facilities and has contributed to an impressive growth and elaboration of the health sciences. Also, it should be recognized that government has supported and strengthened through money, programs, and standards many of these same developments, and now is properly concerned about helping to fill gaps in services arising out of lack of purchasing power or of voluntary initiative. Neither government nor the volunteers should be apologetic about their past performance or potential performance. Now there should be open and free discussion about relative roles bearing on mutual objectives, to avoid unnecessary duplication and assure that no gaps are left between their respective programs.

An important contribution of professional organizations has been made by their initiative and leadership in establishing and maintaining standards for health personnel. The Commission commends those professional organizations which have established mechanisms to develop standards of personnel selection, training, and practice. These standards, formulated by the professions involved, have proved effective in upgrading performance and have enjoyed wide acceptance. Statutory requirements alone are more likely to present "low ceiling" standards than "high floors."

As government involvement in health programs increases, personnel selection needs, training needs, and needs for services will expand manifoldly. Thus, complementary effort by professional groups becomes even more important, and professional organizations should continue their development of such standards and accreditation procedures.

Constructive collaboration in health matters must be enlarged and strengthened at local, state, and national levels among all voluntary agencies as well as with governmental and private elements. The primary attempt throughout should be to enhance the appropriateness, quality, and efficiency of programs and services within the community of solution through the maximum degree of understanding, support, and involvement of the community's citizenry. [M-1]

The Individual Volunteer

Increasingly, at national, regional, and community levels, voluntary organizations and the government will establish many of the necessary working procedures for a modern health partnership. As this comes about, it will underscore the need for a wide and deep involvement of individual volunteers in planning for the solution of community health problems and in acting to carry the plans into operation.

To synchronize the joint approach in the interest of the individual citizen and community is one of the most difficult tasks facing communities. Volunteers are by definition independent; many of them are highly skilled professionals in their specific fields of endeavor who volunteer outside the office in order to "get things done." Many of these people-who-care wear several hats in community affairs, serve on one or more boards of directors, so that at times they are in conflict with themselves when two or more community projects in which they are interested do not mesh easily, or operate at cross-purposes. The situation may be further complicated by the fact that some of the volunteers who donate their time, money, and talents to a specific health or welfare interest also serve as public officials charged with the responsibility of promoting the general welfare.

All of this is part of the American scene — a complex of skills and understanding to be learned by young men and women as they grow in a community and wish to participate in its growth. Voluntaryism has overtones and undertones of business and social status for many people, reflecting a subjective phenomenon difficult for either behavioral scientists or politicians to assess. However, subjective or not, to achieve action a community must secure the interest, the support, and the participation of its citizenry and some agreement among them on priorities for action.

Such voluntary citizen participation is one of the most dynamic resources available in a democracy. Its nurture is vital and its results overwhelmingly beneficial — as indeed the Commission has found in its own undertakings. The very roots of the Commission lie in citizen responsibility. Its initiative was voluntary, its operation has been a blending of private and governmental elements, as has been its financing. Its task forces and advisory committees are made up of leaders from both public and private organizations, each acting in his individual capacity. The Commission's community action studies epitomize the joint approach and the voluntary citizen role.

The 1965 Forum

The Commission's commitment to voluntary citizen participation as a practical and constructive use of resources was demonstrated concretely by the 1965 National Health Forum. This undertaking in cooperation with the National Health Council was a reaching-out to representatives selected by the communities of the nation to test the preliminary findings of the task forces and the community self-studies; in short, to give the members of the Commission a measure of the pulse of America's communities and a reading of the trends and opinions of its leadership — a "listening with an ear to the community."

There were in actuality four Forums — in San Francisco, Chicago, Atlanta, and Philadelphia. More than 200 individuals attended each of the regional forums as active participants in the discussions, for a total of nearly 1000 participants. Each was invited to attend because a committee made up of residents of his area knew of his demonstrated interest and competence in the health field in that region. Of the total, 595 persons were primarily engaged professionally in health services (physicians,

administrators, nurses, dentists, sanitary engineers, and others),
while 258 listed their primary professions as outside the health
field. These included representatives of business and industry,
education, civic organizations, elected officials, government staff,
the clergy, labor, urban planning, communications, welfare, and
others, who were among those providing leadership in conducting
community activities related to the delivery of health service.

Eight hundred fifty-three members of the forums submitted
written reactions to 113 preliminary recommendations presented
by the Commission task forces. The primary purpose of the data
was to provide members of the Commission, in making their
recommendations, with a concept of the regional and total reaction of groups of knowledgeable citizens vitally interested in the
improvement and expansion of quality health care. In addition
to the discussion of specific recommendations, five issues relating
to community health action-planning had been identified through
the community self-studies as issues of major importance; these,
too, were submitted to the forums as discussion topics.

Forum Reactions

If interest and concern can be measured by the volume of
response, of the five issues raised by the community self-studies,
the need for community planning elicited by far the greatest
interest at each of the four regional forums. In descending order,
response indicated interest in the need to improve personal and
community attitudes toward health and health services; concern
over the fragmentation of health services, coupled with fear
that independent action might be curtailed; need to make statistical data available through modern methods of data processing,
in order that data can be effectively utilized; and the need to
develop manpower that can provide leadership within communities for action programs.

To anyone attending the forums, it was obvious that the ivory-
tower or theoretical approach to the provision of comprehensive
health services becomes more and more subject to individual
interpretation the closer one comes to the problems of individual
communities, their customs, and those who form their leadership.
However, in terms of planning, it is evident that new ideas are
widely accepted in relation to the changing concepts of exactly

what geographical areas, authorities, and needs comprise a community. The forums agreed that modern planning for health services must be done on a regional or health trade area basis, and that the planning area should be "commensurate with the size and nature of the problem" — that is, the community of solution. It was acknowledged that broad planning for development of the community in all fields is more complicated than categorical planning in the health field, but it appears that people are becoming aware of the need for total planning in today's society, if the health of a community is to be improved. The forums reflected an acceptance of the need for both long- and short-range planning. Some participants indicated that hospital planning should be conducted only within the context of total health planning in the health trade area.

In accepting the planning need, however, these men and women who have helped to develop the health services now in existence are aware of the danger that the planning process itself — like the services currently available — may become subject to some of the same faults. Forum participants were distinctly concerned that planning bodies might spring up in such numbers that they, too, would be reluctant to cooperate, coordinate, and share responsibilities.

The degree of authority and control necessary for planning groups was hotly contested and the reactions were split. On the one hand, there were proponents of centralized planning bodies with legislative authority to implement decisions, or with at least enough leverage to induce action. Others, however, stated that it is not feasible to legislate this kind of community coordination. The debate here was joined on the efficacy of persuasion versus sanctions, as a community plans to improve its health services. Although the methods to be used in planning were debated, there was agreement that planning had to include not only analysis and exploration, but also application and evaluation.

There was also an expression at the regional forums of something that has been plaguing local administrators of such national programs as the antipoverty efforts: namely, that in today's community planning, the consumer of health services, of all social, ethnic, and economic categories should be involved in the planning that will affect him if the health services are to be both effective and coordinated. How this is to be achieved is one of the major methodological discussions of modern America, but generally, the forums agreed that it can only be achieved if education, communication, and the interpersonal relations of consumers of health services and the providers of those services are given explicit attention.

The contrasting and complex living conditions existing today in the United States were made vividly evident as representatives of huge metropolitan health communities met with people who live and plan in small communities. For the "metroplex," there was expression of the fact that interdisciplinary groups from such cities as New York, Philadelphia, Chicago, Boston, and Los Angeles might be assembled to work out the method for study, action, and evaluation in such complex interlocking and overlapping areas, in order to utilize available resources as well as to plan for new ones. The smaller communities, on the other hand, although still protective of their traditional feelings of autonomy, indicated growing awareness that they must rely on regional and statewide resources if their health services are to be efficient and effective. The cross-currents in such discussions run not only wide but deep. The nation lacks adequate, competent personnel to staff the planning program in most communities on a regular, continuing basis.

In addition, the participants were concerned that communities are not training enough of their own people to provide leadership. In many cities and towns, a young man or woman traditionally learns community leadership by joining a fraternal or service organization and "going up through the chairs" as he contributes to civic betterment by degree. The forum participants indicate that no longer is this enough; that schools should strengthen curriculums in leadership training and community organization long before the college level. They also suggest that the skills and knowledge of public health and social work should be integrated, and that state health departments should strengthen their capacity to assist communities in their planning efforts by developing a staff of community consultants, or by developing pilot programs for leadership training, especially among residents of the smaller communities. Persons who have retired from their regular jobs and persons whose primary interest does not relate to the traditional health and helping professions represent community resources that are not being adequately utilized. There was general agreement that planning for health services can be effected at the community level only if private enterprise becomes interested, as well as government and that top civic leadership ("the people who can get things done") must be involved.

On the assumption that planning can go forward effectively if it is firmly established and supported by the community power structure, the forum participants turned to public attitudes toward health and health services. Here the community leaders agree with national leaders: that health education is the key to improvement of attitudes toward both personal and environmental health. Repeatedly, the discussions centered on the need to develop increased research in the behavioral sciences, so that more can be learned about man's motivations in order to improve the education of both children and adults concerning health. More also needs to be known about ways in which persons of several social and economic groups can work effectively together. There are fewer and fewer communities in which most of the residents share a common ethnic, educational, social, and economic heritage, while for most people in the United States the daily world is one of action, interaction, and reaction among peoples of differing languages, cultures, values, and desires. Persistently in the discussions, two places were identified toward which the new and improved educational techniques toward health should flow: the schools, from kindergarten on; and in offices, industries, or wherever men and women spend their working hours.

Health organizations, as well as individual persons, need to improve their attitudes and relations, the forum participants stated, and their feeling was summarized by one group when it reported its belief that "The solution of community health service problems is possible only if the consumer and the provider of such services are willing to seek ways to reduce the emotional factors that prevent each from accepting the other's faults and virtues in reaching common objectives." These "emotional factors" are at times a strength and at other times a weakness of the voluntary health agencies which have served as the core of the helping services in this nation for so long.

The forum findings were of great value to the Commission in its evaluation of the proposals of its task forces and community studies, and the whole Conference process reinforced its conviction about the importance of voluntary participation in developing health services.

The Commission recognizes the diverse nature of the health programs and services of this nation. Government, private business, and voluntary associations all contribute to the health system. Public and private elements are mutually interdependent. The work of government and voluntary organizations is particularly enhanced by the degree of voluntary citizen participation involved in their processes and services.

A central factor in the growth and development of this nation's high levels of personal and community health has been the participation of individuals and voluntary associations through dedicated leadership, financial support, and personal service. The extension of this tradition of voluntary citizen participation will be essential in guiding the development of community health efforts and in providing important elements of service. [M]

The central question remains: How can the unique resource of the independent citizens of each community be embraced in a new and dynamic concept of voluntaryism? The Commission's task forces and community studies repeatedly draw attention to the vital role of voluntary participation. The Commission recommends action in three areas: the extension of voluntary citizen participation, the enhancement of interagency collaboration, and the application of standards of accountability and performance.

Extension of Voluntary Citizen Participation

Energetic and persistent efforts to extend both the quantity and quality of voluntary participation of individuals and groups is a primary need in the evolving effort to improve community health services. The objective should be the utilization of the full resources of the community in planning for and carrying through the solutions of community health problems and the providing of community health services. This is based on no simplistic notion that all wisdom resides in Main Street or arises from sylvan glens. Rather it is simple recognition that action to mitigate today's health problems requires the informed involvement and participation of the individuals and institutions which comprise the problems and finance the solutions.

Organizations which involve volunteers — including voluntary agencies themselves, some labor groups, businesses, and particularly civic groups such as the women's and service clubs — are and have been undertaking efforts to improve the extent and competence of their volunteers. These efforts should be continued and expanded, and at the same time should be examined and evaluated in light of emerging needs. Such efforts, in the view of the Commission, should be carried forward by the various individual agencies within their own programs and, to the maximum extent, jointly with other agencies.

In the further development of voluntary participation, special attention should be given to three areas: better utilization of talents and competencies, involvement of all social strata and occupational groups, and more effective recruitment and training for policy-making, direct services, and fund-raising. [M-2]

The health partnership must look to leadership development as a challenging issue now as well as for the future. It was quite evident in the presidential campaigns of 1960 and 1964 that young people (far younger than the age of the usual health agency board member) were vitally and passionately concerned in the elections. The same young, eager people can be attracted to voluntary health agencies if they are given challenging roles and an opportunity to contribute to program planning. Some voluntary health agencies are in ruts and an influx of new young leadership could help revitalize them. If, for no other reason, boards of directors and community leadership must look to them because they have voting power and numerical strength. The composition of national health conferences and of boards of voluntary agencies often do not mirror these facts of population.

Occasionally an organized young group takes over the reins of a voluntary health agency, operates it to the benefit of the community, and continues to serve. For the most part, however, the well-adjusted young people who are the product of our high pressure and high education society go through too lengthy an apprenticeship before being invited on to the policy-making boards of health agencies. As high schoolers they operated car-washes for good causes or served in hospitals as "candy-stripers." At middle age, they serve on boards. But, in between, these young men and women — passionately eager in partisan politics either in protest or in defense — are for the most part lost to the voluntary health movement. Voluntary health agencies, in self-examination, should consider the inclusion into their policy-making of influences from two groups of these young people: the well-adjusted, well-educated, and well-fed young men and women who have recently reached voting age and who care vehemently about anything that touches them personally — and, in the same towns and the same communities, the young men and women whose background and experiences give them first-hand knowledge of the problems health agencies are attempting to solve.

Through the new generation, the voluntary health agency may find a means for development within the public-private health partnership that can be just as exciting as was the time a woman's organization established the first "well-baby clinic" in yesterday's century.

Selection and Training

The vitality of community health services is fundamentally dependent on the enlightened participation of volunteers; hence the need for more effective selection, orientation, and training for policy-making, direct services, and fund-raising.

Many of our nation's voluntary agencies have an enviable record for selection and imaginative orientation of volunteers. Too frequently, however, the process is one of chance and default — particularly with respect to selection. Often it is further marred by inadequate inservice training and failure to recognize that the transfer of skills is not always direct.

From the business community, for example, the hospitals, pre-payment plans, and voluntary health agencies have drawn substantial sustenance and support. Contribution of important sums of money, however, does not necessarily qualify an individual for leadership. (Neither should it exclude him!) Nor are social status and dedication to a cause enough. Voluntary citizen participation should be a force for mutual communication. It represents a sharing of talents for problem-solving. It benefits not only the agency directly served but also the individual.

Standards of Accountability and Performance

Many voluntary health agencies were originally organized by small groups of volunteers interested in solving a specific problem. Some developed from local beginnings to become national in scope. Others were established first on a national scale and were then accepted within communities. In recent years, the agencies themselves and members of the public who contribute money to them have been searching for effective methods to review and report on how the agencies spend the funds contributed to them.

The growth of the voluntary health agencies and the amount of money contributed to them by individuals, corporations, and foundations place a responsibility upon their management at all levels to report fully on program, performance, and financing. The need for this kind of accounting to the public is underscored by the fact that private contributions continue in increasing amounts to finance the nation's health programs, even as government allocations to the "health bank" grow.

Within American democracy, government has evolved a system of checks and balances among its separate branches that tends to provide challenge and to stimulate performance, resulting in accountability. Some such system of accountability is necessary for voluntary agencies, including those concerned with health.

It has become increasingly important that there be periodic review of all voluntary health agencies, local, state, and national, by outside, objective, and competent groups, selected by each agency, to insure that programs are continuously adapted to meet changing conditions and needs. [M-3]

The spirit and atmosphere of voluntary support in the United States is a unique and valuable part of our tradition. It is important that all measures be taken to preserve this atmosphere. The complexity of the network of voluntaryism in the United States, the phenomenal increase in public giving, and the general lack of accurate and complete information about some agencies' financial operations have contributed to an atmosphere favorable to the occasional practice of fraudulent activities by unscrupulous groups. Such occurrences have forced governments to act. Laws to control the solicitation of funds from the public have been enacted in some form by more than half of the states. These are positive contributions for the common welfare that merit wholehearted support. The responsibility of government, however, is simply to preserve and insure an atmosphere in which voluntaryism can flourish. Such state laws should be, therefore, not onerous or restrictive in any way, but specifically designed to establish and preserve a climate of voluntaryism. All states should enact and enforce basic reasonable legislation to control solicitation of funds from the public for charitable purposes. [M-4]

The National Health Council issued in 1965 a publication entitled *Viewpoints on State and Local Legislation Regulating Solicitation of Funds from the Public.* This publication served as a useful guide for a number of states in enacting or modernizing legislation in order to include the appropriate responsibilities for government.

A set of "Standards of Accounting and Financial Reporting for Voluntary Health and Welfare Organizations," delineated in 1964 by the National Health Council and the National Social Welfare Assembly, were designed to cover national health agencies and their affiliates as well. Recommendations have also been made paralleling the national standards proposed for state and local agencies. The National Health Council is putting into practice criteria for membership which stress not only fiscal accountability, but also organizational structure and administrative process.

It should be noted that responsible national voluntary agencies participated in the development of standards of accounting and financial reporting, have adopted these standards, and are working toward their implementation. Such agencies constitute a sizable proportion of the membership of the National Health Council, which has established other criteria of organization and management, and have supported this effort. They have a sincere interest in improved standards and fairly conceived and administered accreditation procedures.

The National Health Council should accelerate its efforts to develop and evaluate standards of organization and management, fiscal accountability, and program performance for national voluntary health agencies and their affiliates, leading toward a program of accreditation for agencies, including recommendations for state and local application. [M-5]

Our Governments Are "We," not "They"

The concept of "Partners in Progress" is a sophisticated idea mixing concepts of rigid uniformity and sensitive flexibility — of tax funds and voluntary funds — of the use of voluntary coordination as well as legal licensure. It balances imaginatively long held American traditions.

It contemplates the need for strong organization of voluntary agencies to match strong official health departments. It may involve expenditures of government funds through voluntary agencies as well as government agencies when this results in economy and efficiency, a strengthening rather than a duplicating of resources. It rests, in the last analysis, on an active citizenry participating in many ways. In this government "by the people and for the people," each individual has the opportunity to influence public policies about health services. Our governments are "we," not "they."

Parents participate by planning for and securing comprehensive health care for the family and guiding the health education of their children; friends contribute by helping in time of illness, particularly by being sensitive to the emotional components of ill-health and supportive of the individual when support is needed. As responsible individuals, all can contribute by keeping abreast of and being guided by current professional concepts of how to maintain good health, secure preventive services, and, in the event of illness or disability, how most effectively to cooperate with the health care team to facilitate treatment and rehabilitation.

Individual citizens, in their jobs and vocations, may contribute to community health through industrial health programs, control of environmental health hazards, and promotion of improved services. As volunteer groups, joined together with others who have similar interests in health or in some particular facet of health, individuals may work with national, state, and local voluntary health agencies; with advisory groups to national, state, and local government agencies; or with voluntary non-profit hospitals and prepayment plans. They may also participate as members of civic and fraternal groups, many of which (for example, Rotary, Lions Clubs, Junior League, and Jaycees) have a strong interest in health.

Volunteers, individually or in association, communicate warmth and concern to a person who needs help or information, or simply a listening ear when he is frightened, ill, or alone. As today's society seems to become more impersonal, more crowded, and more complicated, this need is undoubtedly growing rather than disappearing. Voluntary citizen participation in health affairs, whether through government, education, private business, civic organization, or the direct involvement of individual volunteers with specific agencies can and should continue to provide the place, the professionals, and the volunteers who can hear a man out, and respond, when he asks for help.

CHAPTER X

Action-Planning

The idea of planning for change, so that change will occur as directed rather than as the result of haphazard reaction, has become generally accepted in the United States today. We have come a long way since the days of President Franklin D. Roosevelt's first "brain trust," when public reaction indicated that many people thought that planning was, at best, contrived or sly, and, at worst, downright subversive. Until quite recently, however, much of the planning for political or social purposes has been rather fragmentary. Many planners have been professionals who surveyed a single situation, made their recommendations, and went on to other tasks, assuming no responsibility for the actions proposed. Furthermore, a residue of fear persists that planning implies outside control accompanied by loss of independence within the plan's jurisdiction. Although many individuals, institutions, and communities have come to accept the need to plan as an essential base for community endeavor, until the last few years, planning was considered, by and large, something to be entrusted to professional planners.

In many communities today, planning for health has become in actuality a do-it-yourself process involving many persons outside the health professions as well as those within. One of the most significant phases of the Commission's work — the Community Action Studies Project (CASP) — involved 21 communities across the nation which undertook self-studies of their health services.

CASP set about, early in its existence, to discover how planning and action could be linked as parts of the same process and to build into the planning process mechanisms to assure that action would be forthcoming. Action did indeed result, and impressive improvements have been made in health services now available to citizens in the 21 cooperating communities. In view of the demonstrated usefulness of action-planning a discussion of the process is included here.

The Community Health Action-Planning Concept

The nature of today's society and the complexities of health and other community services require a broad approach to planning and action which can be fitted to each particular community situation, yet is in harmony with broader trends and is capable of further development and change. Planning is an action process and is basic to development and maintenance of quality community health services. Action-planning for health should be communitywide in area, continuous in nature, comprehensive in scope, all-inclusive in design, coordinative in function, and adequately staffed. [N]

If communities are to succeed in correlating their health services to provide for the needs of all their residents, they must conceive of planning as an action process. The planning does not end when the facts are in and the report written. The important work of the study is the action which results from and accompanies the gathering of the facts. So persuasive is this hypothesis and so encouraging are the findings of the communities that the Commission recommends that each community (that is, health and medical service area) develop and maintain an action-planning mechanism for health. [N-1]

Action-planning should be *communitywide in area*. Often this area will encompass several towns, counties, or even states, depending on the nature and extent of the problem and the resources necessary to deal with it effectively. It should be *continuous in nature*. Continuity and follow-through are requisite to translating plans into action. It should be *comprehensive in scope*. The CASP analysis especially emphasizes the relationship of one aspect of community health to another, and the interrelatedness of health with the total social, educational, and economic enterprise. It should be *all-inclusive in design* — a partnership between private, voluntary, and governmental sectors representing all elements of the community. Representation should not be confined to health groups; it should include consumers as well as providers of services, civic leaders, and, importantly, health professionals. Experience in the 21 communities shows the value of using these varied representatives responsibly in activities that fully utilize their interests and skills.

Action-planning should be *coordinative in function*. An objective is to attain coordinated action-planning which will eliminate or prevent undesirable overlap and duplication of health services and responsibilities. This does not imply a merging of agencies and groups, but, rather, a concentration on voluntary, coordinated planning in which community goals, priorities, and plans of action are voluntarily achieved through effective citizen and professional involvement and participation. Primary concern should be with programs and action to meet real needs, and not with the idea of a monolithic institution, either private or public.

Finally, action-planning groups should be *well staffed*. Staffing is the key to effectiveness of action-planning. The staff should be comprised of those who know the community, have skills in community organization and community development, know health content or have access to expertise in specialized subject areas, and can effectively collaborate with the professional and voluntary personnel responsible for management and action.

Responsible participation and involvement of all sectors of the community, coordination of efforts, and development of cooperative working arrangements are fundamental to effective action-planning. Health service objectives can be met through processes which provide opportunities for citizens to work together to understand, identify, and resolve problems, to set intermediate and long-range goals, and to act to achieve the goals.

By such cooperation and joint effort on the part of their citizens, communities will find that there is less likelihood that groups will be working at cross-purposes and more likelihood that the total effort will be well coordinated. Achievement of a united effort is important for attaining desirable health objectives. In order to secure the full benefit of their planning activities, communities should utilize appropriate means to achieve coordination of health services. These means might include education, persuasion, financial restraints, or regulations to secure essential coordination. [N-2]

These ends will be realized if an effective dialogue is kept going among community agencies and citizens, and all understand the health goals toward which the community is moving. Each community needs to develop a coordinated health education and communication system. The system should include an interchange of information and ideas between and among agencies and groups, mutual support and coordination of educational activities, and dissemination of general information to the public through maximum utilization of mass media and educational facilities, including the public and private school systems. It should encompass a central health information service for the community which is free and accessible to individuals, families, and organizations via telephone or in person. The responsibility for establishing such a community resource might be shared by voluntary health agencies, professional associations, local health departments, school health councils, and other groups. [N-3]

This endeavor should also bring the educational resources of the community to bear on community health action-planning through voluntary coordination of educational activities within the community. In addition, it should act to stimulate research, demonstration, and innovation in the action-planning process.

Effective planning for health services requires dependable long-range financing to translate plans into action and to sustain those innovative processes which communities may devise for their unique health service requirements. Voluntary agencies, industry, foundations, and government should provide finances for experimentation with new methods of action-planning to effect coordination among health services, improvement of quality, and an increase in their quantity, availability, and acceptability. [N-4]

It is recognized that methods for developing, and money to support, innovative procedures designed to improve community health services are available, but neither in kind nor amount adequate to need. Often, however, sources of help are not known to citizen groups anxious to shore up the health structure of their communities. The federal government and state governments, as well as private professional organizations, can and do provide counsel and funds to help well-authenticated community health enterprises. Given an acceptable objective for which aid has been authorized, federal grants, on a project or matching basis, can be obtained; help is also available from state health departments. Communities should explore all avenues to resources they require. In turn, state, regional, and national agencies and groups should facilitate local community health action-planning efforts in every way possible. They can do so by assisting communities with data collection, analysis, and interpretation, and by providing information from state and regional sources; in other words, data on health, population, economics, labor, and finances. They can often provide expert technical consultation to communities on various aspects of community health services, on study procedures, and on important implementation methods. Too, they can provide skilled manpower to assist in local action-planning efforts when and where needed, and especially in those sparsely populated areas not having sufficient staff. They can assist in recruiting and training action-planning personnel by providing scholarships, by operating personnel placement bureaus, and by supporting in-service and on-the-job training for open-end careers. In summary, they can encourage local innovation, demonstration, and research through the provision of funds, personnel, and consultation. [N-5]

Not infrequently the reason why communities are not fully aware of available resources can be found in an unfortunate lack of coordination of and cooperation among existing health-planning groups. As health-planning activities have gained momentum and scope, a schism between planners themselves has become increasingly apparent. Professional planning staff has come, in general, from two disciplines — social work and the health professions. The two groups have frequently experienced difficulty in communicating and cooperating because of their somewhat different backgrounds. The health planner oriented toward social work tends to be dominant in the volunteer sector, particularly in community health and welfare councils. Health-trained planners are concentrated in the governmental sector and in areawide hospital planning agencies.

The two groups are largely products of graduate schools of

social work, public health, or hospital administration. They turn to different professional organizations and journals for leadership and stimulation, and, as an apparent result, become substantially isolated from each other. In communities, this is evidenced in a strange dichotomy in planning that is more accidental than deliberate. In many communities, separate highly respected professional groups, each with deep conviction as to their responsibility for community health planning, pursue their planning programs with minimum participation from the others. Exceptions to these generalizations can be pointed out readily but they are not sufficient to provide an effective communications bridge for the interaction that would meld the particular strengths of the groups and produce the mutual respect and confidence so essential to true collaborative effort.

Because effective health planning must recognize the need for a full governmental voluntary partnership, the viewpoints and skills of planners from social work, public health, health and welfare councils, and hospital administration must be brought together to produce a professional cadre of the highest possible caliber. Toward this end, schools of social work, public health, and hospital administration and graduate schools of social and political science and public administration should initiate or expand short-term and long-term health-planning courses to provide opportunities for public health personnel, social welfare personnel, and hospital planners to be trained together with the broadest possible professional orientation and communitywide perspective. [N-6] Further, steps should be taken to encourage schools of public health, social work, hospital administration, and public administration to develop a suggested core curriculum for training health planners. [N-7]

The concept of planning as an action process recognizes that planning for community health cannot and should not be isolated from other needs of the community. Each civic function requires specific approaches relevant to specific situations. Whatever the objective of planning, and however widespread the participation of all sectors of the community in it, constructive results cannot be assured unless the planning group has access to and understands the facts and their implications for individual and community health. Facts are elusive — often distorted by prejudice, often inaccessible, often of unmanageable dimension. Building a case for health services on inadequate or undigested data is a hazardous business, likely to provoke justifiable citizen nonsupport of a worthwhile service or facility that has been projected on the basis of insecure data. To avoid such false starts, the Commission recommends that each community develop capabilities for collecting, analyzing, and using data for action-planning with the cooperation and assistance of appropriate state or regional groups.

Local health departments and health institutions working with professional societies and community health action-planning groups should assure the development of capabilities for obtaining the data necessary for realistic and relevant goal-setting and action-evaluation. Resources for continuing data collection and analysis should be identified, related, utilized, and strengthened as necessary. Personnel with training and competence in data analysis and interpretation should be brought into the action-planning efforts at the very outset. [N-8]

Approaches to data collection differ as resources and capabilities in each community differ. The self-study planning guide developed by the Commission can be used as an illustrative framework for constructing a system in which relevant data can be collected for problem identification and evaluation. Sharing information by several agencies within a community is essential.

Health-oriented groups may not be able to sustain a data collection and analysis operation by themselves and will need to look to alternate resources. As automatic data processing systems are developed at state and regional levels, explorations should be made for sharing of data pertinent to local action-planning operations.

Full utilization should be made of all available sources of data: such as records, reports, vital statistics, and survey data. However, in many situations planning can proceed with facts or information available from well-informed persons living in the area. As the prominent civic leader of one of the studies said, "action, in my opinion, is far more likely to occur with respect to reasonably attainable goals set by well-informed people, even though they are not wholly expert and some of their 'data' are no more than an intelligent sense of smell."

The Community Action Studies Project

Thousands of citizens who have participated in grass-roots planning during the past three years have discovered how to bring about a new kind of citizen participation which has significant implications for improving the quality of living. Action-planning is such a process. It helps citizens make social decisions that will bring results. It is an educational experience which encourages participants to identify and analyze facts, set goals, resolve conflict, obtain action, and evaluate achievement. Learning the techniques of this process is extremely valuable since the evidence suggests that basic deficiencies are a lack of information and understanding, lack of participation and involvement, and lack of personal identification with community needs and interests. Action-planning is personal, geared to each community and its people. Because communities and people differ, their goals of achievement differ. The process must take these differences into account in order to deal with them in a realistic and relevant manner.

To test planning methods and to stimulate communities to take effective action to improve health services five basic study activities were developed: self-studies of community health services by 21 communities across the nation; study of the dynamics of community action, utilizing the technique of process analysis; a retrospective examination of community health studies and their implementation; a study of factors contributing to the readiness or unreadiness of communities to act; and a series of special case studies of episodes that were reputedly successful in the field of community health.

Community Self-Studies

From the first public announcements of the formation of the Commission in 1962 through April 1964, 131 communities in 45 of the 50 states indicated varying degrees of interest in conducting a self-study. Of the 21 communities selected, 4 represented communities with populations in excess of 500,000; 11 were in the 100,000 to 500,000 population range; 6 were communities of fewer than 100,000 persons. They represented all nine United

States Bureau of Census regions and a variety of climatic, cultural, and economic settings.

Approximately 8,000,000 people were affected by decisions, plans, and actions taken in these 21 communities. All studies were organized, staffed, and financed through local initiative. The Commission assisted the studies with consultation, process analysis, development of self-study guidelines, and conferences for study leaders. Limited consultation was available to communities in the process of study and in the technical aspects of their health problems. Periodically, study leaders from the communities assembled to exchange ideas for their mutual benefit and, at the same time, to give the Commission information on which it could evaluate the processes and techniques of community action-planning as they evolved.

Through these procedures, the studies provided two distinct but complementary types of information: from the community point of view, information vital to solving actual local health problems; and, from the standpoint of the Commission's work, information on the relative values of various processes of planning and action which might be applied by other communities.

Although all aspects of achievement had not been accounted for at the time this Report was prepared, available results confirmed that it is possible and feasible for diverse groups within communities to collaborate to identify problems, seek solutions, resolve conflicts, and improve health services. Civic and professional leaders demonstrated that they can work together within their own community, gain the support and cooperation of governmental and private agencies, and enlist the cooperation of health departments as well as other agencies whose primary concerns are not those of health.

In fact, the whole self-study enterprise stands as an affirmation of community self-reliance and an indication of what other communities in the United States could do in their own health interests — self-reliance awaiting discovery. Wherever they are, such reservoirs of persons willing to accept responsibility should be tapped for purposes of providing citizens with desirable health services. Community action-planning groups should, therefore, seek to increase research, demonstration, and development of new approaches, especially in health education, data collection and utilization, methods of implementation of action-plans, and organization of community health services. [N-9]

In organizing their objectives, study communities looked both toward long-range goals and to immediate or short-term objectives. The achievements of action-planning had already been demonstrated as early as one year after goals had been established. In one community, laws and practices for admitting the mentally ill to institutional care had been changed; in another, hospital and allied facilities were being expanded, while medical residency and medical research programs were being developed simultaneously. In this same community a $15,000,000 bond issue was being proposed to finance development and expansion of a medical complex, $10,000,000 of which was for outpatient services, extended care facilities, laboratory services, and other programs designed to improve personal health services.

At least three communities were developing areawide health departments. Two of these communities were scheduled to vote to decide on the establishment and financing of a health department. One community was acting on a 2.5-mill tax levy as provided by state law. One group had improved pediatric services by augmenting these services in existing facilities, thereby eliminating a plan for a separate hospital. Another community was developing a mental-health-oriented human relations center. An environmental health rural renewal league was under way, giving priority to housing, water supplies, and waste disposal. Still another community had decided to fluoridate its water supply. One community had stimulated the enactment of several state health statutes, including the merger of policy-making units of the health and welfare departments. A one-cent sales tax for health, welfare, and education services had been voted by a four to one plurality in another self-study community, half earmarked for health and welfare, half for education. Another community group, after identifying school health program needs, had taken direct action, resulting in administrative action by the Superintendent of Public Instruction to improve the school health program, bringing it in line with study recommendations.

One of the tools developed by the Commission to aid communities in organizing and conducting health studies was a self-study guide. The CASP adapted the APHA *Guide to a Community Self-Study* for use by study leaders. After its use in actual operation and subsequent field modification, a new *Guide* was developed, based on these field experiences. It is designed to help communities identify their health problems and solve them.

Primarily action-planning for health is local — almost by definition because there is where health services are delivered and received. But local operations and systems necessarily relate to and interact with state, regional, and national systems and resources — public, private, and voluntary. Usually the community's first intergovernmental tie is with the state, and all states should be equipped to extend the kinds of help discussed in this chapter. Each state should use its State Health Policy and Planning Commission to effect health action-planning in the state. Community health action-planning will be of substantial value in developing statewide health plans. These statewide plans will, in turn, contribute to, and form the basis of, national health planning.

Communities which at first were defensive found that, by using outside consultative resources, local groups were able to define their problems, decide what they wanted to achieve, and get action within a relatively short period, while still maintaining their local autonomy. Another continuing result of the community studies is that they have started a chain reaction. As other communities became aware of the action-planning experiences of the 21 self-studies, requests have increased for information on processes, methods, experiences, and assistance.

Process Analysis

While the 21 communities held themselves up to the mirror, another CASP program examined the dynamics of community health action-planning in order to identify the important factors in the process. The one question central to the research activity was: What patterns of community organization promote an effective self-study of health needs and stimulate action addressed to those needs? Using five university-based teams of social scientists, this research effort was developed as a part of the CASP program and was called "process analysis" since the task was to analyze the processes of community action. Several conclusions emerged.

The single most important one has to do with the ability of the person staffing the action-planning project — the self-study co-ordinator. The staff coordinator works at the joining-point of social forces, the point where national interests, professional experience of health consultants, the desires of the study's initiators, and the thrust of professional and civic community interests converge. As the title implies, this person is charged with co-ordinating the many interests, ideas, and local traditions into a workable blend of activities. This finding is so significantly important that community health action-planning groups must give increased attention to recruiting and training persons to enter the health field, particularly persons to handle staff functions for assessment, planning, and action. A second major conclusion was the significance of the selection of citizens who are aware of and are willing to accept the responsibilities that the study will demand. Another conclusion was the importance of scheduling a practicable, step-by-step study process.

It would seem obvious that effective leadership and logical organization stand out as prime requisites in effective community health action-planning. But the analysts point out that the chances for the success of the self-study are better where economic, political, and professional leaders involved in the study know one another and have collaborated to good effect in the past. They already command the respect of other leaders and can mobilize public opinion and obtain participation by other competent and busy people — especially the young, tomorrow's community leaders who bring a special kind of unfettered commitment to community action. These community leaders are apt to be members of boards of private health agencies and are often advisers to public officials. Through their influence, public and private agencies can be brought to collaborate in health action-planning.

At one time or another, in all 21 studies, the comment was made that nonhealth issues are always closely interrelated with health issues. So by actual experience community residents have learned that problems associated with population growth, urbanization, automation, and industrialization, as well as politics and economics, are problems related to health.

Even in this mobile world, people are innately suspicious of outsiders, but the 21 studies found that persons and groups from outside the community brought positive influences to bear on the studies. The Commission helped in some instances to stimulate the initial decision to undertake a study. In others, it served to build morale, as the individual communities, by sharing problems and ideas with their counterparts in other study communities, became aware that they were a part of a national effort both to improve health services and to discover how best to go about achieving that improvement. Other outsiders, who quickly ceased to be considered as such, served as consultants, while communities worked out methods of organizing, conducting, and obtaining action on their studies and resulting recommendations. Technical consultants helped groups to set goals that were realistic, relevant, and feasible within their specific community.

Above all, the study communities emphasized that it was wasteful and inefficient to think of action-planning as a "some-time thing." There must, they agreed, be some sort of continuing mechanism for planning in the community, so that individual leaders, separate agencies, and related community groups, assembled to achieve specific cooperative projects, would not drift away to other interests or return to operative isolation. Continuity of education in the process, they also found, was fundamental to the whole concept of individual and community responsibility for action. Their experience indicated that programs of communication and education must be continuous in order to increase awareness of the values of health, health needs, and available health services and to shape attitudes toward health that will influence individual and community behavior in achieving health services of high quality for that community.

Community Readiness Study

When the Commission began its community studies, one condition for acceptance of a community in the study project was that it be ready, willing, and able to conduct a self-study with no major barriers in sight that might inhibit the effort. Some communities were obviously unable to meet this requirement. As a result, the Commission initiated research to find out what makes one community ready for such a study, while another is not.

The Community Readiness Study's preliminary findings indicated that the "unready community" may be characterized as one which has no effective mechanism for planning, not only in areas of health but in education, industrial development, or other aspects of social and economic life. In this community, action comes as the result of crisis and is therefore unplanned and improvised under conditions of urgency and emotional, if not physical, stress. In the "ready community," where planning is an established habit and is supported by community leaders, officials are able to anticipate many crises before they arise. Even if a critical event is unforeseen, the resources of the community are more readily marshalled for an orderly reaction.

In a feasibility study, conducted in the state of Oregon and financed through a special PHS research grant, further inquiry was made into the dynamics of community health planning with special reference to community readiness to plan and act on a variety of health and other civic problems. Three elements were identified as being essential: citizen readiness, leadership readiness, and presence of an effective planning mechanism through which community energies can be channeled. In the unready community, one or more of these three factors is missing.

A flow model of readiness, then, can be visualized:

Leadership readiness
Citizen readiness
} Planning mechanisms → Community plan of action → Community action → Individual treatment or prevention

This study reinforced conclusions drawn from the self-studies by showing that citizen awareness and leadership awareness are interrelated with the operation of a planning system; no one factor by itself is sufficient to spark community action. Certainly, the mere study of health problems is not sufficient to produce readiness for action.

Retrospective Analysis

To dig further and to find out why so many health studies have not, in the past, resulted in action proportionate to the investment, the Commission took inventory. Community health studies are conducted at about a rate of 265 a year in this country. Although CASP's retrospective analysis, based on a sample of 447, was incomplete after this report went to press, some observations can be made.

In the main, health studies conducted since 1955 have examined large communities in populous regions, in centers where the average income and educational level are high and where health and welfare expenditures are about three times the national average. Although health planning involves change and potential controversy, retrospective studies showed that a few communities have faced up to potential controversy and dealt with it forthrightly. A few with abundant resources found ways to increase efforts in using those resources to supply health services. Nevertheless, normal inertia and a distaste for controversy are formidable obstacles.

Often pertinent health data on a community are not readily accessible. Frequently, the form in which data are available is not standardized for ease of use or comparison and, at times, the data themselves are unreliable. This research confirms the finding that community health services contain a number of competitive systems which by their individuality deny to themselves the uses of a joint fund of information. One common and recurrent theme is the need to coordinate existing services where they are wastefully duplicated. Some communities are developing autonomous planning councils to achieve this coordination.

Two significant findings have emerged thus far from the retrospective analysis. First, variations in communities, in their problems, and in approaches to resolution of them must be recognized. Action-planning should develop different patterns, rather than suggest a single model to encompass all communities. Second, since much has been said about how to study health problems, but little about how to get action, implementation must be emphasized throughout the action-planning process.

The CASP investigation, pursued as it was on an across-the-nation basis, disclosed the need for leaders to marshal community resources to improve health services. These reservoirs-of-readiness can be energized if the resources of state universities and private institutions of higher learning are made available to communities to facilitate community health action-planning. [N-10] The processes of action-planning are several and flexible, as they should be. No *sine qua non* has been developed yet nor is one likely, or even necessarily desirable. Even though evidences of success are reassuringly clear, there is still need for continuing experimentation and research.

Special Case Studies

Case studies in selected communities that were reputedly successful in action-planning provided additional insight into factors leading to success or failure. Common denominators observed include several which, when grouped together, apparently provide the profile of a successful planning community that achieves action.

First, an effective program is often identified with one or more strong personalities. These figures lead, push, cajole, raise pertinent issues, face up to controversy, stimulate discussion of the issue, and precipitate the kind of political situations wherein people must take positions, defend them, resolve the conflict, and make decisions. Second, the successful program is likely to be in a community where there has been a long, carefully built tradition in community planning. Third, success is likely to be associated with cooperation between public and private sectors, and civic leadership plays a significant role in either sanctioning or vetoing proposed programs. Finally, it appears that the successful community knows how to deal aggressively with conflict and controversy by rational discussion, *quid pro quo* compromise, respect for majority opinion, and whatever other means are effective in reaching a decision. Without this sometimes agonizing confrontation of disparate interests and points of view, resulting in decision for change, a community endeavors futilely to freeze the status quo. In such instances, the situation frequently deteriorates because community wounds caused by unresolved controversy usually defy suturing.

Citizen action to improve health services is not new in this country. We accept as our birthright participation in political parties and support of and from voluntary associations of all kinds. What we have tended to lose in our expansion and specialization of health services is the effective involvement of people in decisions that affect their health. It is a loss we can ill afford. Action-planning for health services offers the opportunity to regain it. The future demands that the opportunity be grasped now.

CHAPTER XI

The Future

There is in the year 1966 a sense of urgency throughout the land wherever people gather to talk about health and the delivery of health services.

During the four years in which the National Commission on Community Health Services has been at work, the attitudes surrounding this sense of urgency have changed. Where once the persons concerned with improving the health of individuals and their environment concentrated on the idea that we *must* do something, today these same persons, joined by thousands of newly interested community leaders in many fields, are saying, "we *can* do something." In effect, this entire document is a report on the needs to be met in the future and a discussion of some of the ways in which these needs can be met. Yet what has been accomplished is only a beginning. What next? What of tomorrow?

Tomorrow is separated from today by only one night, but tomorrow also stretches to the end of every man's life and beyond. In predicting the future of health care in the United States, then, it is logical to state the social and economic trends of our times as they relate to health services and the recommendations on which agreement can be reached. Some needed changes can be achieved in a relatively short period of time; others will take longer. It takes only one jump to cross some chasms, but others are so wide and deep that they cannot be jumped and instead must be bridged, a girder at a time.

With the adoption during the 1960's of health legislation of unprecedented scope and importance, coupled with the marked increase of local community interest in improving health services, the foundation for future development is now firmly based on a public-private partnership for health. Health services within communities and among them are extremely uneven, so that some areas must work to solve the most elementary of problems while others, having met their basic health needs, are concerned with the expansion of quality services, well integrated and available to all residents. But, for all communities, at whatever stage in development of health services, the traditional dialogue about government and private funds, government and private facilities, and varying levels of governments has taken on new dimensions.

The tide of change on which we are swept into the future must involve the entire health partnership. For it is now evident that neither the public nor the private sector of the American community can achieve the delivery of health services alone. For this reason, planning for health and implementation of the plans will go forward more effectively and more swiftly if the various components of the health industry give up their separatist attitudes in favor of collaboration. This premise must be accepted if the nation is to meet its present health problems. Those of the future will be even more demanding.

The population of the United States will soon pass 200,000,000 with an increase to 210,000,000 in prospect by 1970 and about 250,000,000 by 1985. Approximately one-half of all the residents of the country will be living — by 1985 — in three huge metropolitan complexes: Boston-New York-Philadelphia-Norfolk; Milwaukee-Chicago-Detroit-Cleveland; and San Francisco-Los Angeles-San Diego.

There are 18,000,000 persons over age 65 in the nation, and this year, under terms of Medicare, they will have the ability to pay for most of their health services. Since the over-65 population will reach a total of 25,000,000 by 1985, health services must be expanded rapidly to meet the demands of this group. At the same time that the older group within the population is increasing, the projected birth rate indicates that the median population age in 1980 will be about 25 years as contrasted to the 1960 population mid-point of 30 years. Additionally, the proportion of women in the population is increasing, with an expected ratio of 75 men to 100 women among those over 65 by 1970.

No one can today predict with certainty the eventual impact of Medicare and population change on health services, but it

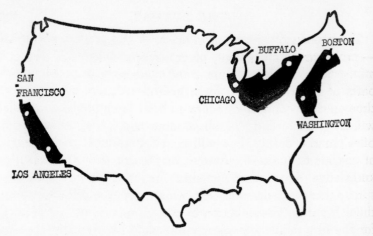

Figure 4. The three areas which by 1985 may contain half of the population of the United States.

can be estimated in some degree by the realization that in the first year in which the Medicare provisions of Social Security come into operation, the federal government will spend an additional $3,200,000,000 for health care. Other medical programs provided for in the same statute will add another half billion dollars. The national ability to pay for health care is being further improved through the growth of private health insurance, provided in a variety of prepayment plans. Some 70-77 percent of the civilian population, excluding those in institutions, now have some degree of hospital coverage.

As the economic, social, and educational opportunities of the American people improve, more of them will become aware of health benefits; more will demand them; and, in a population that is growing, the need for health services will also grow.

What kind of health services will this population need and demand? Within each individual's knowledge and perception, he will seek services that improve the quality of his life. The American of tomorrow will expect to have access to the kind of treatment he needs, in community-based facilities where treatment services, emergency services, and preventive services can be adapted to his individual needs. As the fruits of an affluent society become more evenly available to the population, the task confronting the persons who plan, operate, and deliver health facilities and services will continue to increase in size and diversity.

The process of urbanization brings both benefits and problems — problems of movement, of crowding, of overlap, and of administration. Early retirement and increased leisure will become parts of the way of life for a greater number of people. With time on their hands and money in their pockets, these Americans will fly more aircraft, purchase more boats, drive more automobiles. In the doing, they will continue to add to the pollution of the air and water resources of the country; and, as general knowledge about environmental health hazards continues to spread, they will demand that community health services control these hazards. The direction of public opinion in health matters for the future has been clearly indicated by events of the recent past. For example, today it is common knowledge that clean air must be available for cities quickly, by whatever methods are found to be efficacious.

As the Commission completes its studies, it is obvious that the ferment of American concern about its health services is rising to the top of the national consciousness. Based on the health services which present scientific information and technology now made available, there is almost no limit to future achievement if the enlightened self-interest of the public continues to develop.

Let us, then, look forward to the profile of community health services in the United States for the next ten to fifteen years. The health professions and the allied health personnel have not been idle in continuing their search for knowledge and for adequate utilization of that knowledge.

In delineating its responsibilities within the public-private partnership, the Public Health Service plans to provide support and guidance in directing the thrust of research where the needs are greatest. Such a program is designed to bring cohesion and continuity into the huge national health research effort in the allied health sciences. Emphasis is also being given to converting science into practice by helping to channel new knowledge through private medicine, hospitals, universities, and governmental agencies of all kinds for the benefit of the consumer of health services. There will also be rapid development of new patterns of administration and delivery of health services.

Private funds probably will continue to be the major financial resource in the development of health facilities and health manpower. But, because of the size of the need and the celerity with which facilities must be made available and personnel must be trained, the federal government is moving rapidly toward increased support in both these critical areas. With private medicine and with public and private agencies and institutions in every facet of the health field, the government will almost certainly cooperate to improve standards of service and quality of care. The trend toward increased federal financial support and influence upon community-based health services is reflected in Congressional action.

Central to future development of the public-private partnership is the manner in which the efforts of health personnel are organized to provide health services. The report of the Commission emphasizes its primary concern in recommending that all individuals have a personal physician who is the integrating and continuity factor in comprehensive care. The conditions and forces working against such an achievement are great, but the need is overriding and must be met.

The growth of specialization in health services will undoubtedly continue, as will the increasing variety of health personnel. As the population continues to congregate in huge metropolitan areas, the trend toward large, regional health centers will also continue. As communities organize their health resources in more integrated constellations of services, there is danger that the consumer, while receiving quality care, may be lost in the impersonalities of efficient operation. This already occurs to some extent, and one of the greatest challenges of the future, for all health personnel, is to treat the entire population while providing personalized care of high quality for each patient. The search for the answer to this difficult problem rests with the medical and other health professionals themselves, as they redesign their curriculums, the peripheral limits of their interlocking responsibilities, the organizational structures through which they work, and their attitudes toward community service in the broad sense.

Through the increased use of automation in hospitals and laboratories, through high-speed collection, storage, and dissemination of data on patients, disease, research, and community characteristics, it may be possible that the physician, the nurse, the social worker, and others within the modern health team can be freed from detail to give more personal service to patients.

Increased efficiency in the use of resources must be achieved if health services are to be made available and accessible to every resident and are services in which he has confidence. To-day's health services have faults, but American medicine on the whole can and does provide quality care; its challenge in the immediate future is to devise means to expand and extend its already great abilities. Meeting the health services challenge will require the continuous pressure of an alert and articulate public, aware of its needs, of the extent of its resources, and of the type of organizational structure needed.

It has always been one of the human ironies that men gain knowledge more easily than they learn to use it. Knowledge about health is no exception. Discoveries in the chemistry and physiology of the human mind indicate that personalities can be significantly changed. Scientists have broken the genetic code; they have developed artificial organs of the body; rehabilitative medicine has made great strides. Without doubt, the future of health services will include further knowledge of utilization of the findings of such research. Science will continue to explore methods of intervention for shaping life before birth, to change psychological and physical characteristics and conditions during life, and to extend the length of life. As this is achieved, the en-tire environment must be improved so that the life we lead will be worth living. This brings any projections toward the future heights of health back to the most immediate of tomorrows — to the individual community, the present state of its health services, and its capacities to effect change.

In the past, most of the health services available in any American community were financed and provided by the men and women who had always lived there, had personal and finan-cial roots and interest in the community, and expected to be buried there. However, although America used to be called "the great melting pot," communities were not always homogeneous, and health care, being a very personal thing, was organized along personal lines.

It was from these beginnings that the voluntary "health hierarchy" of the last 150 years became an important part of the community "establishment." Churches, lodges, and brotherhoods often owned their own hospitals and dictated their admissions policies. In similar fashion, voluntary boards of directors administered policies of voluntary health agencies and voluntary health programs, many of which were organized to control a specific disease. That part of the community power structure concerned with health services has ordinarily been made up in great part of the older leaders in the area. Usually, they inherited their positions of leadership from other members of the same social or religious groups; their power was based on dynasty and ownership. Typically, health agencies, and hospitals as well, have been "agency centered" rather than "community centered" in their programs and policies.

One of the changes which can be predicted is a change in the community health services power and dynasty, which has already begun to make itself evident. In part, it is a further extension of the public-private partnership, but several other factors are equally important. Within each community, the base of power is moving to a different group of individuals. Many of them are newcomers; their families were born elsewhere; they, themselves, do not necessarily feel the community permanency of their forebears. These newcomers come into a community quite often as representatives of large industries, trained in the new techniques of management. Their power rests on interpersonal relationships and the use of a range of managerial and administrative information and technique which has come into widespread use and acceptance only within the last few decades.

Civic participation provides many rewards to the volunteer, the most important of which is probably personal satisfaction. It is also a means by which a newcomer can achieve status in a community, and industries encourage their middle-management group to be active in local voluntary agencies. One result of this injection of "new blood" into agencies may be that individual board members of hospitals and other health agencies may look beyond the specific needs of their own organizations toward a sharing of broader community responsibilities for the community health services system. Such a trend must be supported if comprehensive personal and environmental health services are even to be approximated.

The positions and recommendations presented in this report

are all directed toward the attainment of the goal of comprehensive personal and environmental health services in each community. In one form or another, they have been discussed and debated at length by the Commission task forces, by the self-study communities, by regional forums, and by a wide range of other health organizations. As a part of the ferment of concern about health services, they have been the subject of an unprecedented "talking treatment."

Progress in the implementation of these recommendations lies in rational health planning and policy formulation at all levels — local, state, and national — and most crucial in the implementation is that action must take place in local communities. Communities, therefore, have a basic decision to make in the immediate future. They must decide to what extent they will develop continuous programs of action-planning for comprehensive health services and how much they will depend on crisis planning based on sporadic needs.

A preview into this portion of the community future for health is available in the results of a questionnaire to which all 21 of the communities participating in the Commission's Community Action Studies Project responded in December 1965. Results of the studies will be presented in a Community Action Studies Project report, but some of the insights gained by communities in these self-studies should be here indicated as signposts for the future.

The original goals of the community self-studies were similar in nature, regardless of the size of the community. The communities were searching for means to coordinate services and programs; develop new awareness and concern about health problems in a wide segment of the population to achieve a broader base for support; develop planning mechanisms to encompass and serve a regional or multijurisdictional area; develop a public health department or greater support of the existing department; and develop specific services in such areas as mental health, environmental health, expansion of health facilities, and recruitment of manpower.

Some of the studies are still in progress, but events occurring in the months following the establishment of the study goals indicate that the study leaders, who were the motivating forces behind the organization of the study groups, were aware of the problems and needs which later emerged from the study efforts.

One of the major accomplishments resulting from the studies was a better informed citizenry, including the people actually involved in the study, as well as the general public itself. Repeatedly, these comments indicate that through the involvement of many people in the study process, communities achieve a recognition of health needs, a realization of the inadequacies of health services and, through this critical awareness of need, secure additional cooperation between and among community groups.

Although each community encountered its own specific issues and resolved them in its own way, all of them faced to some degree such problems as the conflict and controversy reflecting apprehension about the aims, goals, and reasons for the study; the issue of communitywide planning; struggles for power and influence; and an apathy or lack of interest among some.

The apprehension was partially caused by what some of the agencies and groups — both public and private — perceived as a threat to home rule or agency autonomy. This was apparent in some communities in voluntary health agencies and in local health departments in others. Where the need for such a study was not universally accepted, there were disagreements; in some instances, the individuals involved in the study group had misunderstandings about their roles.

The basic question raised by the issue of communitywide planning centered on the question: Who should plan for health services in a community? There was also resistance to planning itself, the reluctance of some agencies to share data, and a question of public and private relationships and agency responsibilities in the community planning process. We can anticipate a continuation of these problems. In many ways, the future will be not unlike the present. In the struggle for power and influence, personality conflicts will emerge, political interests and citizen acceptance of some of the recommendations will continue to be an issue, vested interests will pose problems, and political fears about the effects of bad publicity from health problems will be very real in some communities.

It is in the means through which the study communities set about clarifying and resolving these conflicts that lessons will be learned by other communities for future studies. First of all, the study leaders of the future must recognize that the conflicts are real and that efforts to resolve them will require tact and persistence. Not all the conflicts will be resolved, but, in most instances, study leaders will use one or all of three major methods used by the community self-studies. A political process of assembling leaders representing divergent views around a conference table to thrash out solutions face-to-face (conferences, meetings, personal contact, and thorough discussion) will continue to be a major factor. Personal persuasion, ranging from "tactful handling by the chairman" to personal explanation by persons intimately involved in the study to others who are suspicious and apprehensive, will continue to be useful, but it will require patience and continuing effort. Public information media will be a prime means by which purpose of the studies can be explained to the public.

Significant in its implications for future community ability to improve health services is the realization in many of the study communities that — even though they wish to protect their local autonomy — they can no longer "go it alone" in providing many of the necessary health services.

The accent on action-planning is an integral part of the community self-studies of the Commission and has major relevance as a concept in future improvements of health services. Too often, the group which studied a health problem in past years either did not or could not implement its recommendations. This failure can no longer be tolerated, for the needs and the opportunities are currently so great that a study without resulting action is now a luxury communities can no longer afford.

It is extremely difficult to pinpoint cause and effect in chronicling the major events related to the health services of the nation in the early 1960's. The formation of the Commission itself was a national indication of the extent of interest within the health professions and the voluntary organizations, professional societies, government, private foundations, and industry. The establishment of its task forces, its community studies, and its National

Health Forum which provided sounding boards for both professional and citizen expression on most of the problems and their possible solutions.

At the same time, other groups, organized to probe specialized segments of the health problem, have been at work. The health legislation adopted by the 88th and 89th Congresses and espoused by two Administrations is a reflection of the force of public demand for more and better health services. The Social Security Amendments of 1965 (Medicare) provide for the funding of health services for important groups of individuals, particularly the elderly. The Clean Air Act, as amended, provides funds for research and development of air pollution controls, but it also, significantly, provides a timetable for that development and enforcement. This is also true of the Water Quality Act. The Community Mental Health Centers Act of 1963 and its 1965 Amendments provide a means by which a variety of combinations of public and private sponsors can finance the construction and staffing of community mental health centers. The Heart Disease, Cancer, and Stroke legislation of 1965 offers an opportunity for collaboration by medical schools, medical centers, hospitals, and other treatment facilities to pioneer in the next round of research, training, and treatment utilization to benefit the victims of disease. Between November 1963 and May 1966, 20 federal health statutes of major significance were signed into law; their implementation is under way.

Simultaneously, interest in international health has grown and has become an important element in the implementation of economic and social development programs. Part of this concern is the result of international awareness that health hazards of the nuclear environment cross boundaries. But much of the concern for international health has little or no relation to the hazards of the nuclear age. These are concerns about people in their usual living situations. Famine is "usual" for some; malaria is "usual" for others. The results of international health efforts cannot today be estimated in precise terms; however, if health services in this nation are uneven, the gaps in most other parts of the world are so wide as to be catastrophic to mankind, unless the quality of living is brought into closer balance.

While the scope of the Commission did not include international problems, it is felt that, if the recommendations are found to be useful and effective in the United States, they will have their effect on the work of international health agencies and on other national health programs as they emerge. The Commission is concerned that its efforts be continued by appropriate groups and that ways be evolved by which its studies and recommendations can be given practical application.

At a time when the genetic code has been broken, when men and animals orbit through space for weeks in the completely artificial environments of self-contained vehicles, when it is not unusual to catheterize and visually explore an artery for a suspected aneurysm, the American community should not be victimized by its own lack or organization of available health resources. The Commission is convinced that in the United States no citizen need go without the full range of services for health in his community if he is willing to assume, with the community, the responsibility to plan, work, and pay for it.

CHAPTER XII

Positions and Recommendations

From the wealth of fact, study, and discussion which resulted from two and one-half years of study by six national task forces and 21 community self-studies, the Commission has formulated 14 positions or statements of conviction, and a series of recommendations which stem from them. These positions and recommendations, on which the preceding chapters were based, are brought together here both as final summary and basic substance of the report. They are stated without interpretation, and reference is made to those earlier pages in which they are discussed and elaborated.

POSITION A: HEALTH SERVICES AND JURISDICTIONAL AREAS

Political considerations raise problems not specific to health affairs, but crucial as the setting for health action. The most significant political issue in community health organization is that of revision of outmoded, overlapping, and ambiguous jurisdictions. Health service administrative areas must be efficiently functional in terms of major health problems and can no longer be circumscribed by traditional community, state, and national boundaries.

The organization and delivery of community health services by both official and voluntary agencies must be based on the "community of solution" — that is, environmental health problem-sheds and health service marketing areas, rather than primarily on political jurisdictions. [Pages 4, 129]

RECOMMENDATIONS

A-1. Each state should have a State Health Policy and Planning Commission, responsible to the governor, which would advise him on health planning for the state. Such a Commission would be representative of governmental, private, and voluntary groups. It would have no administrative functions, but would, by the plans it made, set the framework for administration of health services in the state whether these services were offered by governmental, private, or voluntary groups. A major function of this Commission would be to examine, with the state health department, the state's pattern of health jurisdictions and recommend groupings of one or more political units as regions: problem-sheds for environmental health services or health marketing areas for personal health service. [Page 130]

A-2. Regions, based on communities of solution, should be established as organized units for administration of health services. They should correspond to geographic areas from which communities can draw every needed service. Each region should have available an adequate supply of every health skill and resource. In addition, regions established for personal health services should have a fully equipped and staffed medical center.

Both providers and consumers of health care should participate in the development of regional plans, and every community or rural area should be included in one region or another. Reasonable attention should be given to the established trend of patterns for health care, as well as to traditional political boundaries of cities, counties, and states. Boundaries of the regions established should be regularly reassessed and revised so that they can be continuously adapted to the changing dimensions of health problems. [Page 131]

A-3. Every region should have a health-planning council, organized on a permanent basis, under top-echelon citizen and professional leadership; financed from a variety of sources; responsible for general health services and facilities planning within the context of the region's total spectrum of health services; and coordinated with the planning of other community, regional, and state agencies, especially the State Health Policy and Planning Commission. [Page 131]

A-4. Regions and communities should take appropriate interim measures to help pave the way for the planning councils. One step the Commission urges is cooperative interagency planning — governmental and voluntary — of service programs and facilities, in such manner as to assure joint utilization of those services and facilities. [Page 131]

A-5. Where the "community of solution" of a health problem requires coordinated action by several jurisdictions, appropriate use should be made of compacts, agreements, and/or interstate authorities. [129]

A-6. Through participation in and assistance to international efforts to control disease and raise standards of living, the federal government and the voluntary agencies and societies (such as the national voluntary health agencies through their international counterparts, the American Medical Association through the World Medical Association, and the National Citizens Committee for the World Health Organization) should help to protect the health of citizens in all communities of the United States. [Page 6]

POSITION B: COMPREHENSIVE PERSONAL HEALTH SERVICES

All communities of this nation must take the action necessary to provide comprehensive personal health services of high quality to all people in each community. These services should embrace those directed toward promotion of positive good health, application of established preventive measures, early detection of disease, prompt and effective treatment, and physical, social, and vocational rehabilitation of those with residual disabilities. This broad range of personal health services must be patterned so as to assure full and intelligent use by all groups in the community.

Success in this endeavor will mean much change. It will require the removal of racial, economic, organizational, residence, and geographic barriers to the use of health services by all persons. It will require strengthened and expanded licensure and accreditation of services, manpower, and facilities. It will require maximum coverage through health insurance and other prepayment plans, and extension of such insurance to cover the broad range of services both in and out of hospitals. Finally, success will require a citizenry that is sufficiently well informed and motivated to follow established principles conducive to good health, and to cooperate fully with health services in all phases of prevention and treatment of illness and disability. [Page 17]

RECOMMENDATIONS

B-1. Communities by deliberate planning should develop patterns of comprehensive health services of optimum quality and assure their availability, accessibility, and acceptability to all. This comprehensive approach to health must embrace the health needs of all age groups from the very young to the very old. It should include a full range of health services — health promotion, including continuing health education, family planning, the broadest array of safety measures, and all environmental health services appropriate to a given area; prevention of disease and disability including immunization, presymptomatic case-finding, and nutritional services; effective programs for school, mental, industrial, occupational, and dental health; early diagnosis and treatment with systematic follow-up as required to achieve maximum physical, social, and vocational rehabilitation. It should make available the necessary continuum of facilities and services, including hospital, nursing home, physicians' offices, and coordinated home care. It should provide for analysis of patterns of sickness and mortality, particularly to identify high-risk groups, and studies of other indexes of the effectiveness of health programs and evaluation of the threats to health implied by social and environmental change, leading to special programs of consultation, advice, and service as needed. [Page 19]

B-2. All persons and agencies responsible for health services should foster the gradual building of an integrated program that will provide comprehensive personal health services of optimum quality, equally available and accessible to all, in each community. Separate systems of health care now exist for many groups in the population such as veterans, labor organizations, merchant seamen, and the medically indigent. The welding of the separate systems into a communitywide program would preclude new construction or expansion of hospitals for separate population groups and the gradual integration of such facilities into total community services. [Page 21]

B-3. Each community should develop an effective counseling, placement, and referral service for patients in cooperation with the health care facilities system and the professions providing health services. [Page 29]

B-4. Concerted action should be taken through law enforcement, legislation, and education to limit the practice of medicine to those who are scientifically educated and licensed. Quality health care should be the goal for Americans. The public should be advised by all possible means and methods that quality health care can be obtained only from scientifically trained practitioners. Health educators, professional organizations, and official and voluntary health agencies must intensify their efforts to inform the public of the hazards to the health and wealth of this nation posed by quack and cult practitioners. A national citizen commission should be established to create a model code for states to adopt to provide for uniform licensure of the health professions. [Pages 67, 68]

B-5. Existing licensing and accreditation procedures for health care facilities and services should be strengthened, expanded, and enforced by appropriate authorities. Accreditation should be extended to include nursing homes, rehabilitation facilities, and noninstitutional services such as home nursing and home care. Hospitals and other institutions and facilities and non-institutional services should strengthen programs to insure that accreditation standards are met by continuing assessment of performance. [Page 30]

B-6. Hospitals and other health agencies should cooperate in the strengthening and development of facilities and services for patients who do not require hospitalization (such as out-patient services, extended care facilities, home care programs, geriatric day centers, and foster family programs) to promote comprehensive personal health care through a network of appropriate alternative settings. [Page 30]

B-7. It should be the responsibility of the community to make rehabilitative services available and it should be the responsibility of all physicians, whether engaged in special or family practice, to utilize these services. There should be increased emphasis on physical medicine and rehabilitation in medical school curriculums, in internship and residency programs, and in postgraduate medical education. Also, programs to train allied health personnel required for effective rehabilitation services must be expanded and funded. The Commission further recommends research and demonstration aimed at providing prepayment coverage for rehabilitation services as the principal way of financing these services for all who need them. [Page 33]

B-8. The application of psychological and social sciences to health should be given increased recognition by the health professions. The importance of environmental stress in the causation and of environmental support in the treatment of psychiatric disorders should be recognized in the organization of general medical, occupational, social, and welfare services. Psychiatric services are needed in varying degree by an appreciable part of those seeking medical care and should be an integral of all treatment programs. In addition, the current national movement toward comprehensive community mental health and retardation services and the great resources in public interest, experience, and money that have been developed should be integrated into community plans for comprehensive health services. [Page 34]

B-9. There should be increased research and demonstration efforts to develop improved methods of organization and delivery of health services and to improve the quality of such services. [Page 37]

B-10. The integrated program of health services should continue to be financed from a variety of sources, including individual out-of-pocket payments, insurance and prepayment plans, and public funds. Health insurance should be developed or extended to cover all persons employed, self-employed, and unemployed, together with their dependents, in order to eliminate financial barriers to medical care. All interested parties should pursue this extension of coverage by all possible methods, including the appropriate use of public monies. Health insurance should cover out-of-hospital care as well as in-hospital care and it must cover the full range of services: preventive, diagnostic, therapeutic, and rehabilitative for both mental and physical illness. [Pages 71, 74]

B-11. Restrictive legislation which forbids or impedes the development of prepaid group practice plans should be removed, and full experimentation with such plans should be encouraged. [Page 73]

B-12. Rigorous examination of all factors involved in setting health insurance rates should be undertaken by the plans before rate changes are proposed and by rate-setting authorities reviewing proposals. These factors include benefits, utilization, controls, provider costs, and the impact of government programs covering selected segments of the population. In order to provide protection for the high-risk subscriber, the Commission favors either community rating or a type of class rating that accomplishes the same purpose. [Pages 74, 75]

POSITION C: THE CHANGING ROLE OF THE PERSONAL PHYSICIAN

Every individual should have a personal physician who is the central point for integration and continuity of all medical and medically related services to his patient. Such a physician will emphasize the practice of preventive medicine, both through his own efforts and in partnership with the health and social resources of the community. He will be aware of the many and varied social, emotional, and environmental factors that influence the health of his patient and his patient's family. He will either render, or direct the patient to, whatever services best suit his needs. His concern will be for the patient as a whole and his relationship with the patient must be a continuing one.

In order to carry out his coordinating role, it is essential that all pertinent health information be channeled through him, regardless of what institution, agency, or individual renders the service. He will have knowledge of and access to all the health resources of the community — social, preventive, diagnostic, therapeutic, and rehabilitative — and will mobilize them for the patient. [Page 21]

RECOMMENDATIONS

C-1. All arrangements for organization or delivery of comprehensive personal health services should be based on a firm and continuing relationship between the individual patient and a personal physician. This personal physician is responsible for bringing the individual into the integrated program of comprehensive personal health services, and for providing or securing needed health care. In order to make the most efficient use of limited physician manpower, health care functions not requiring medical training should be delegated by the physician to other members of the health care team to the maximum extent that is practical. [Page 22]

C-2. The community should provide and the personal physician should utilize a full range of community health services, within and outside the hospital. Every hospital should have a service for personal physicians, and conversely, every qualified personal physician should have a staff appointment in one or more accredited hospitals with privileges in accordance with his capabilities, and each personal physician should have access to a program of continuing medical education. The personal physician should work as part of a team in which the special abilities of the different members are integrated for a common purpose — the health and well-being of the patient. Many of these skills have been available to him in the hospital and other institutions in the past and more will be needed in the future, but there is an urgent need now for the development of means through which he can best use these talents and skills in the home and in connection with other outpatient services. The medical profession should work with community leaders to develop means through which this can be accomplished. [Page 25]

C-3. Every personal physician should maintain an association with other physicians which makes medical service to his patient available at all times, 24 hours a day, 7 days a week. Communities should explore a number of organizational means, ranging from informal associations to institutionalized groups, for integration of personal health services. Emphasis should be given to the stimulation of those forms of association among physicians which would facilitate overcoming undesirable fragmentation of health services, maintenance of high standards of quality of care, and payment mechanisms that reduce economic barriers to preventive services and to prompt diagnostic and therapeutic services. The group practice of medicine, as a specific way of integrating the service of physicians, has demonstrated that it can provide an effective and efficient method of furnishing comprehensive medical care of good quality. Such organization of services should be stimulated and encouraged as one of the best routes toward comprehensive personal health services. [Pages 23, 24]

C-4. Efforts should be begun now to produce the number and quality of personal physicians needed for the delivery of comprehensive personal health services in the decades ahead. This will require a national effort to provide appropriate educational opportunities and career incentives, taking into account the established framework of specialization. Attracting the medical graduate to a career as a personal physician will be possible only if there is general recognition of the importance of his role and he is accorded status, professional satisfaction, and income comparable to that of other physicians.

The program required to produce the number of personal physicians needed will be comparable in magnitude to that which expanded medical research in the past two decades. Large-scale financing will be necessary for support of teachers and trainees, facilities, programs, and educational research. Medical schools will need to alter very considerably their present intramural curriculums, and develop community-based and community-oriented teaching programs as part of the training experience. The education of personal physicians and the attraction of interest of medical students to careers in this area require programs which emphasize continuity of relationship between the physician and the patient and the responsibility of the physician for assuring comprehensive care. The personal physician of the future must have a broader knowledge of all the elements of comprehensive health services than he now receives during his graduate and undergraduate training. His education should place primary emphasis on the development of basic competence in preventive medicine, internal medicine, pediatrics, psychiatry, and rehabilitation. The American Medical Association and the Association of American Medical Colleges should take the initiative in developing specific recommendations for the undergraduate and graduate training of personal physicians. Further, university medical centers should accept responsibility for providing personal health services to a limited but representative sample of the population through a demonstration unit designed for teaching and research on comprehensive health care. The training of specialists will and should continue, but the education of all physicians should include appropriate courses and experience in community medicine.

In view of the complexity of medical knowledge and the speed of change, medical schools should take the initiative in developing programs of continuing education with the cooperation of other groups such as the medical society, hospitals, and the health department. Means should be found to secure for the personal physician status and income comparable to that of other specialists, and the medical profession should give serious consideration to according the personal physician status by the establishment of an appropriate board certification. [Page 27]

POSITION D: COMPREHENSIVE
ENVIRONMENTAL HEALTH SERVICES

Optimum health can be fostered by prospective planning and management of comprehensive environmental health services. This means going far beyond assuring pure water, clean air, and safe food. It means assuring hygienic housing to provide space for adequate privacy and family sociability, for places of rest and quiet, and places for activity and recreation. It means assuring an external milieu for man designed to stimulate his greatest growth potential. [Page 38]

POSITION E: CONTROL
OF MAN'S ENVIRONMENT

Air, water, and land are not unlimited, and the maintenance of these resources at high quality becomes daily a more complicated challenge to all leadership — political, governmental, industrial, business, labor, educational, and agricultural.

The American environment is being contaminated at a rate rapidly approaching saturation and the health of the people is in jeopardy. The need for decisive citizen action is urgent. Moreover, people are using physical, biological, and chemical products indiscriminately, unaware, for the most part, of their hazards.

Improving the quality of our environment requires additional financial resources, public and private, adequately planned and programmed to insure the control of water and air pollution and protective measures against contamination from physical, biological, and chemical products, including the increasing use of radioactive materials. [Page 39]

RECOMMENDATIONS

E-1. Public health agencies should administer those programs where the protection and promotion of health is the primary objective. Where health is not the primary objective and a program is administered by another agency, the public health agency should be responsible for establishing and assuring enforcement of environmental health standards. [Page 40]

E-2. There should be a nationwide, continuous, automated air sampling network including every community that is a potential or known source of air pollution, whether that pollution be biological, chemical, or radiological. Such sampling would provide a basis for the development of prevention and control programs in communities. [Page 43]

E-3. Governmental and industrial funds should be provided in vastly increased amounts to assist in developing adequate research and control programs, but prevention and elimination of sources of pollution must proceed on the basis of present knowledge. [Page 43]

E-4. The federal government should exercise its interstate commerce powers to encourage manufacturers to continue voluntary efforts to improve currently available devices that reduce health hazards from pollution. The federal government, in cooperation with state health and motor vehicle agencies, should require that all motor vehicles be equipped with the most effective means of eliminating the noxious gases from motor exhausts. [Page 44]

E-5. The nation should increase its attack on water pollution. An unprecedented, large-scale effort is required to develop and finance comprehensive water pollution control programs by: eliminating the existing ceiling for the federal sewage treatment facilities grant program; seriously considering a method of financing construction and maintenance of sewerage systems analogous to that used to finance interstate highway systems, with federal sources financing the major portion of the system and state and local sources supplying sewer lines to tie into the main system; and increasing research in new methods of waste disposal and conversion. [Page 45]

E-6. Four basic steps should be taken now to deal with the fast growing problem of solid waste disposal: waste disposal and conversion should be planned and operated on a problem-shed basis; health agencies should establish adequate community standards for collection and disposal of solid wastes, and, in cooperation with the responsible operating agencies, exercise leadership in evaluating the adequacy of these activities; state governments should adopt enabling legislation to provide their political subdivisions with workable legal and administrative tools to perform this function effectively; and industry, foundations, and government should give high priority to research into methods of solid waste disposal and conversion. [Page 46]

E-7. Industry should be required to reduce its pollution of both air and water. [Page 46]

E-8. All federal, state, and local institutions should cease to add pollution to the environment. [Page 46]

E-9. Research by government and industry should be substantially increased to determine the immediate and long-range cumulative effects of radiological techniques, and of physical, biological, and chemical products on man to plan and conduct education and enforcement programs and to keep pace with the new technology. [Page 69]

E-10. Special measures should be taken to teach the consumer to avoid the misuse of physical, biological, and chemical products now available for use in the home, on the farm, and in industry. Protection from such products as solvents, pesticides, plastics, and devices involving the use of microwaves includes labeling to aid in consumer education as to correct storage and use, systematic testing of the products, and continuous monitoring of their distribution where indicated. [Page 69]

E-11. Industry, governments, voluntary agencies, educational institutions, and communications media should join in the development of continuous and effective education programs designed to inform the public of the danger of pollutant activities and the steps to be taken to avoid them; develop easily recognizable signals for alerting the public to the level of air and water pollutants (the smog-level signals now in use in Los Angeles, or the fire-danger levels used by national parks, for example); and publish and dramatize through all media what to do in response to these warning signals. [Page 69]

E-12. The federal government should require manufacturers of pesticides and other economic chemicals to assume the burden of proof that their products are not harmful to human life if properly used. [Page 69]

POSITION F: ACCIDENT PREVENTION

Accident prevention is an integral part of comprehensive personal and environmental health services. Health leadership must increase its efforts to prevent accidental injuries, disabilities, and death. [Page 49]

RECOMMENDATIONS

F-1. The State Health Department should take the initiative in developing statewide accident prevention programs, eliciting the cooperation and support of other official and voluntary agencies. [Page 49]

F-2. The United States Public Health Service should be given funds to establish a national accident prevention, research, training, service, and information facility analogous to the present Communicable Disease Center. [Page 50]

F-3. The present accident prevention efforts of voluntary agencies, associations, industry, and government should be encouraged and be given increased financial support to assess and expand their programs in line with demonstrated needs and modern concepts. [Page 50]

F-4. There should be stricter enforcement of present laws and regulations designed to control or diminish accident hazards. [Page 50]

POSITION G: FAMILY PLANNING

Family planning should be an integral part of community health services. Private and public health agencies must accept responsibility for provision of family planning services and for the support of scientific research on human fertility. Family planning is essential to individual and family health and contributes to a healthy community. All individuals have the right to have convenient access to information about the different methods available and to practice those methods acceptable to them for the benefit of their offspring, their family life, and their community. [Page 58]

RECOMMENDATIONS

G-1. Scientific research on human fertility and on related factors influencing population changes should be immediately intensified. [Page 58]

G-2. Instruction in family planning should be a routine health service carried out in appropriate facilities by qualified personnel. [Page 58]

POSITION H: URBAN DESIGN AND HEALTH

Planning for a healthy environment is an essential consideration in urban design. Immediate steps must be taken by those responsible for the control of land use, transportation, economic development, and related physical and social planning to coordinate their activities to provide for the most effective use of space for our rapidly growing urban population; avoid ill-effects that may be associated with high population densities; reduce hazards to physical and emotional health from overcrowding where it exists; and contribute to an aesthetically and emotionally satisfying environment conducive to positive health.

Nearly three-fourths of our population will be urban dwellers during the last quarter of this century. Some sections of the na-

tion, embracing several states, will soon be broad belts of high population density. The urban center is fast becoming the metropolitan area and several metropolitan areas are merging into the megalopolis. The effects of so many people living so close together need attention now to prevent those factors that contribute to ill health and to foster those that enhance a better health and life. [Page 59]

RECOMMENDATIONS

H-1. Immediate steps should be taken to make the full range of health services of the community (with emphasis on prevention and rehabilitation) available and accessible for those who live in areas which combine high population density, chronic poverty, and deprivation. [Page 59]

H-2. The Department of Housing and Urban Development and the United States Department of Health, Education, and Welfare should take primary responsibility, in cooperation with other appropriate federal agencies and voluntary and professional organizations, for developing criteria to measure the effect of population mobility, density, and urban conditions on the physical, emotional, and social health of people; and in promoting research and experimentation in urban design, land use, and population distribution as these relate to health. [Page 60]

H-3. Model legislation should be developed to require all programs related to physical city planning (land use, urban design and renewal, highway construction, public housing, and so forth) to provide for healthful distribution of population; protection from hazardous, noisy, and unaesthetic environments; the availability and accessibility of comprehensive health and welfare services; and space for recreational and cultural activities. [Page 61]

POSITION I: EDUCATION FOR HEALTH

Education for health is a fundamental aspect of community health services and is basic to every health program. It should stimulate each individual to assume responsibility for maintaining personal health throughout life and to participate in community health activities.

The community has a responsibility for developing an organized and continuing educational program concerning health resources for its residents. Each individual has a personal responsibility for making full use of available health resources. [Page 62]

RECOMMENDATIONS

I-1. State departments of education and local school boards should assume greater responsibility for the development of health curriculums. In so doing, the schools should look to health departments and voluntary health agencies for assistance in providing continuity and resources. [Page 64]

I-2. Health departments and voluntary health agencies should make available resources for health education programs in business and industry. These resources should be utilized to supplement in-plant health information and counseling efforts. [Page 64]

I-3. More applied research in educational techniques and methods should be undertaken to supplement and draw from physical and social science research findings, particularly those which apply to health attitudes, motivation, and behavior. [Page 66]

I-4. Health education personnel should be given courses covering the needs of the rapidly expanding health field, including administration, community organization, and action-planning. [Page 66]

I-5. Schools of public health should maintain a department or unit that specializes in relevant areas of education and communication. Schools of public health and schools of education should cooperate in training health educators. [Pages 66, 84]

POSITION J: HEALTH MANPOWER

Effective utilization of available health personnel will reduce the current manpower shortage, and continuous evaluation of the use of manpower, accompanied by necessary changes and retraining, will provide additional manpower for existing and new health services. However, to provide comprehensive community health services in the next decade will require an unprecedented effort to recruit, educate, and train additional man-

power for the health team. Such an effort should be intensive, planned, and continuous, and should emphasize teamwork among all levels of health manpower.

Every community must have available the skills and techniques of many kinds of health personnel. These needs are increasing in terms of numbers of people as well as kinds of skills required. The wide range of manpower for environmental and personal health services includes not only engineers and physicians, but many varieties of laboratory technicians, dentists, nurses, pharmacists, physical, occupational, and speech therapists, homemakers, health aides, social workers, psychological and vocational counselors, and nutritionists.

To deliver comprehensive health care, all members of the health team must work together, with each member consistently contributing his most highly developed skills and recognizing others' skills and particular contribution to the health of people. They must, at a minimum, coordinate their work. [Page 79]

RECOMMENDATIONS

J-1. The Public Health Service should assume responsibility for collecting and reporting health manpower data on a nation-wide basis, using standardized classifications in cooperation with associations representing health occupations, educational institutions, and voluntary health agencies. [Page 80]

J-2. Additional public and private funds should be devoted to experiments and demonstrations to increase the productivity of all types of health personnel and improve the range and quality of service. [Page 80]

J-3. In order to attract and retain health personnel, wages and salaries should be made comparable to those received by people performing similar jobs in the community. Wage and hour laws and other protective legislation should be amended to include health personnel wherever their place of employment. [Page 80]

J-4. In addition to demographic and other pertinent data, as criteria for determining community health personnel needs, all health agencies should determine the personnel required to carry out their programs effectively by establishing the nature of the problems, the goals to be attained, and the number and type of personnel needed to attain these goals. [Page 82]

J-5. Research in utilization studies should be conducted to delineate the different functions required to meet the needs of patients and to determine the necessary level of training to perform these functions. Many universities and organizations have the resources to perform such analyses and should be supported in this effort. [Page 83]

J-6. Dental schools should assume increased responsibility for training auxiliary personnel with broadened functions and promote their use by example. [Page 86]

J-7. Schools of public health, social work, community organization, and public administration should develop academic programs that will provide qualified personnel to conduct community self-studies. [Page 87]

J-8. Special emphasis should be given to securing and preparing top-level health service administrators for responsible positions of leadership in health. This will entail selective recruitment and training that includes administrative management, economics, sociology, and political science. Health administrators must have professional satisfaction, status, and financial reward commensurate with the importance of their role. [Page 89]

J-9. Concerted efforts should be made to attract secondary school students to health careers by improving counseling, work experience in health facilities, and expanded work-study programs. [Page 93]

J-10. Governmental agencies, educational institutions, health agencies, and professional and occupational groups should undertake positive measures to recruit from part-time personnel, minority groups, the technologically displaced, and the handicapped. [Page 94]

J-11. Those communities and institutions that have eliminated racial discrimination and segregation in the provision of health care should be commended, and such practices should be completely eliminated in the interest of economy, good health care, and simple justice. [Page 94]

J-12. Vigorous efforts, voluntary and governmental, should be undertaken to increase the supply of professional social workers in medical and health services through the construction of expanded and new educational facilities; financial support for faculty field instructors and related costs of teachers; greatly increased scholarship aid through fellowships and traineeships; and research and experimentation in methods of professional education aimed at innovations intended to improve the quality of professional education of social workers for medical and health services. [Page 96]

J-13. Increased training for social workers in medical and health settings, where training is community-oriented, should be provided in concert with other members of the health team. In addition, since it is probable that graduate schools are not going to produce enough social workers to meet the increasing needs in this field, research and demonstration should proceed toward a teaching program to train personnel of less than professional skills to perform limited duties within the health team. [Page 96]

J-14. Qualified candidates for training in a health career should receive the financial assistance they need from government, industry, or other sources — in the form of grants, scholarships, or loans — to complete their training. Further, the United States Department of Health, Education, and Welfare should be provided with funds to support the training of environmental health personnel, through the establishment of environmental research and training centers in universities. [Pages 90, 94, 96]

J-15. Efforts should be intensified to expand accredited nursing education programs which prepare persons to become registered nurses with college degrees, through baccalaureate programs; registered nurses without college degrees, through two-year colleges or hospital diploma programs; and vocational or practical nurses, through vocational school or hospital programs. [Page 97]

J-16. Since the two-year community colleges can play an important role in training auxiliary health personnel, present programs for health occupations in junior colleges should be expanded as rapidly as is consistent with quality. Curriculums in two-year colleges should be designed, insofar as possible, to permit additional education at a later time for those students who want to continue their health career development. Two-year colleges should be aided by: grants from private sources and government to develop training programs for health occupations; federal funds to universities for the preparation of faculty required to teach in two-year colleges; scholarships from private and government funds to students in two-year colleges who wish to prepare for health occupations; and affiliation with four-year colleges and medical institutions that can supply laboratory and clinic experience, as well as consultation and association with health professionals. [Page 97]

J-17. To the fullest extent possible, members of the health team should receive their education jointly in order to give each an appreciation of the goals and skills of the other and practical experience in working together on common problems. [Page 98]

J-18. Educational institutions offering health training should cooperate actively with professional associations and official and private agencies in developing programs of in-service training and continuing education for allied health services personnel. [Page 99]

POSITION K: HOSPITAL CARE

The rapid rise in the cost of hospital care in the past two decades is a matter of grave concern to the American people. The upward pressure on costs results from the development of new and costlier diagnostic and treatment techniques; increases in salary costs as hospital wages become competitive with industry; the increasing burden of educational and training programs in hospitals; and the inability of hospitals to match rising costs with increased productivity.

The Commission takes the position that further increases in hospital costs must not be accepted complacently, but that a wide range of vigorous and persistent actions must be taken by all parties concerned to moderate the costs of hospital care without adverse effects on its quality. [Page 111]

RECOMMENDATIONS

K-1. High priority should be given to the development, in the hospital or affiliated with the hospital, of extended care facilities, self-care units, rehabilitation units, home care programs, geriatric day centers, foster-family programs, and outpatient services to provide a network of alternative services and to encourage appropriate utilization of facilities. [Page 106]

K-2. There should be established, within the framework of regional or state hospital associations, groups — composed of trustees, medical staff, and administrators — that could promote a broader outlook and serve as information sources and forums for exchange of ideas. [Page 109]

K-3. Those responsible for the education of hospital administrators should emphasize that understanding the health community of which the hospital is a part and relating the hospital effectively to allied health care facilities and programs are basic to success as an effective administrator. [Page 110]

K-4. Hospitals and allied facilities should explore every available additional means for improving management, increasing efficiency, and reducing cost. Such means should include systems of joint management — laundries, laboratories, drug formularies, and purchasing services — and exploration of the possibility of merging small hospitals. [Page 110]

K-5. There should be programs of research and demonstration grants to hospitals, councils, universities, and other organizations to support studies of hospital operating costs and capital financing, as well as pioneering programs aimed at cost reduction. [Page 111]

K-6. Regional health-planning councils should be responsible for initiating or coordinating health facility planning for the region. Such councils should be provided with sufficient authority to assure coordination of equipment, space, staff, and utilization of facilities within its jurisdictions, as well as authority to review and evaluate plans for new facility construction or change of function. [Page 113]

K-7. Third parties — health insurance plans and governmental agencies — should reimburse the hospital for services rendered at full current cost. [Page 114]

K-8. Research should be undertaken to determine the net cost of educating interns, residents, medical students, nurses, and other allied professional and technical personnel, and to determine the appropriate sources of funds for meeting those costs. [Page 115]

K-9. Communities should experiment with pilot projects and demonstrations to test specific procedures to achieve maximum efficient use of facilities. [Page 116]

K-10. Priority should be given to construction of extended care facilities under voluntary, nonprofit auspices, physically or functionally related to a general hospital. [Page 116]

POSITION L: ORGANIZATION, ADMINISTRATION, AND FINANCING OF OFFICIAL STATE AND LOCAL HEALTH AGENCIES

Every state should have a single, strong, well-financed, professionally staffed, official health agency with sufficient authority and funds to carry out its responsibilities. The state should assure every community of coverage by an official health agency and access to the complete range of community health services.

This state agency must be able to work effectively with federal agencies, to provide all the environmental and personal health services for which it is responsible, to stimulate and support the development of local health units that will provide official health agency services to local communities, to take leadership in broadening the scope and quality of health services available to its communities, and to respond positively to the health needs of the public.

This single agency, in which all the major health programs of the state government should be concentrated, would be able to coordinate the various environmental, preventive, curative, and rehabilitative components into a comprehensive health service system. It should be responsible for setting the health standards of other state programs even though they may be a secondary activity of another agency. [Page 139]

RECOMMENDATIONS

L-1. States should take steps to effect the consolidation of their official health services (including mental health, school health, mental retardation, the administration of medical care programs for the indigent, and the medical aspects of rehabilitation in a single state health agency. [Page 140]

L-2. The state should assign to its health agency responsibility for developing and maintaining all programs necessary to protect people from environmental hazards and from poor quality health services, and it should be specifically charged to initiate action to meet new and changing health needs. [Page 140]

L-3. Each state should secure for its health agency sufficient financial support provided in the most flexible manner possible, with proper safeguards. [Page 140]

L-4. The state health agency should stimulate the development of local health units to provide coverage for local communities. The local unit may be responsible for a city, county, city-county, or several counties combined, depending on the configuration which can best serve the community effectively and efficiently. It should carry out duties delegated by the state and such other functions as are locally determined, recognizing that such agencies are most likely to be effective in responding to the needs of the community as they arise. These local health units should be adequately financed and staffed with full-time personnel who have been especially trained in the public health sciences. [Page 141]

L-5. The state should delegate as many of its functions to the local health unit as can be properly and effectively carried out within the community concerned. [Page 141]

L-6. Financial support for local health units should be expanded. Local governments depend on the state for their power and responsibilities; therefore, the state has an obligation to see that local units are adequately financed. Increased state aid should contain financial incentives for any necessary reform in structure and organization of local health agencies, including appropriate consolidations and regionalization. The federal government should assist in financing community health services through the states by awarding grants in as flexible a manner as possible, consistent with the maintenance of standards of quality. Categorical project grants should be employed only to assist in solving specific serious health problems currently needing special emphasis; categorical formula grants should be reviewed periodically as to accomplishments and phased into the basic grant when the categorical approach is no longer justified; and the basic (general) formula health grant should be increased both absolutely and as a proportion of total grants. [Page 142]

L-7. General support funds for research should be made available to public health departments by the federal government. They should be provided with the intent of furthering the advance of the total research capacity of the health department, including employment of competent research personnel. [Page 147]

POSITION M: VOLUNTARY CITIZEN PARTICIPATION

The Commission recognizes the diverse nature of the health programs and services of this nation. Government, private business, and voluntary associations all contribute to the health system. Public and private elements are mutually interdependent. The work of government and voluntary organizations is particularly enhanced by the degree of voluntary citizen participation involved in their processes and services.

A central factor in the growth and development of this nation's high levels of personal and community health has been the participation of individuals and voluntary associations through dedicated leadership, financial support, and personal service. The extension of this tradition of voluntary citizen participation will be essential in guiding the development of community health efforts and in providing important elements of service. [Page 160]

RECOMMENDATIONS

M-1. Constructive collaboration in health matters should be enlarged and strengthened at local, state, and national levels among all voluntary agencies as well as with governmental and private elements. The primary thrust throughout should be to enhance the appropriateness, quality, and efficiency of programs and services within the community of solution through the maximum degree of understanding, support, and involvement of the community's citizenry. [Page 154]

M-2. Energetic and persistent efforts should be carried forward to extend both the quantity and quality of voluntary participation of individuals and groups as a primary means of utilizing the full resources of the community in planning for and carrying through the solutions of community health problems and providing community health services. Present efforts to extend voluntary participation should be examined, evaluated, and strengthened. Special attention should be given to better utilization of talents and competencies, involvement of all social strata and occupational groups, and more effective recruitment and training for policy-making, direct services, and fund-raising. [Page 161]

M-3. There should be periodic review of all voluntary health agencies, local, state, and national, by outside, objective, and competent groups, selected by each agency, to insure that programs are continuously adapted to meet changing conditions and needs. [Page 163]

M-4. All states should enact and enforce reasonable basic legislation to control the solicitation of funds from the public for charitable purposes. [Page 164]

M-5. The National Health Council should accelerate its efforts to develop and evaluate standards of organization and management and fiscal accountability and program performance for national voluntary health agencies and their affiliates, leading toward a program of accreditation of such agencies, including recommendations for state and local application. [Page 165]

POSITION N: ACTION-PLANNING FOR COMMUNITY HEALTH SERVICES

The nature of today's society and the complexities of health and other community services require a broad approach to planning and action which can be fitted to each particular community situation, yet is in harmony with broader trends and is capable of further development and change. The Commission believes that planning is an action process and is basic to development and maintenance of quality community health services. Action-planning for health should be communitywide in area, continuous in nature, comprehensive in scope, all-inclusive in design, coordinative in function, and adequately staffed.

The responsible participation and involvement of all sectors of the community, coordination of efforts, and development of cooperative working arrangements are fundamental to effective action-planning. Health service objectives can be met through processes which provide opportunity for citizens to work together to understand, identify, and resolve problems, to set intermediate and long-range goals, and to act to achieve the goals.

The readiness and ability of communities to respond to health needs and problems are dependent, in large part, on the presence of effective mechanisms for planning. [Page 168]

RECOMMENDATIONS

N-1. Each community (that is, health and medical service area) should develop and maintain an action-planning mechanism for health. [Page 168]

N-2. To secure the full benefit of their planning activities, communities should utilize appropriate means to achieve the coordination of health services. These means might include education, persuasion, financial restraints, or regulations to secure essential coordination. [Page 170]

N-3. Each community should develop a coordinated health education and communication system. The system should include an interchange of information and ideas between and among agencies and groups, mutual support and coordination of educational activities, and dissemination of general information to the public through maximum utilization of mass media and educational facilities, including the public and private school system. It should encompass a central health information service for the community which is free and accessible to individuals, families, and organizations via telephone or in person. Responsibility for establishing such a community resource might be shared by voluntary health agencies, professional associations, local health departments, school health councils, and other groups. [Page 170]

N-4. Voluntary agencies, industry, foundations, and the government should provide finances for experimentation with new methods of action-planning to effect coordination among health services, improvement of quality, and an increase in their quantity, availability, and acceptability. [Page 170]

N-5. State, regional, and national agencies and groups should facilitate local community health action-planning efforts in every way possible. They can do so by assisting communities with data collection, analysis, and interpretation, and by providing information from state and regional sources, that is, data on health, population, economics, labor, and finances. They can often provide expert technical consultation to communities on various aspects of community health services, on study procedures, and on important implementation methods. Too, they can provide skilled manpower to assist in local action-planning efforts when and where needed, and especially in those sparsely populated areas not having sufficient staff. They can assist in recruiting and training action-planning personnel by providing scholarships, by operating personnel placement bureaus, and by supporting in-service and on-the-job training for open-end careers. In summary, they can encourage local innovation, demonstration, and research through provision of funds, personnel, and consultation. [Page 171]

N-6. Schools of social work, public health, and hospital administration, and graduate schools of social and political science and public administration should initiate or expand short-term and long-term health-planning courses to provide opportunities for public health personnel, social welfare personnel, and hospital planners to be trained together with the broadest possible professional orientation and communitywide perspective. [Page 172]

N-7. Steps should be taken to encourage schools of public health, social work, hospital administration, and public administration to develop a suggested core curriculum for training health planners. [Page 172]

N-8. Each community should develop capabilities for collecting, analyzing, and using data for action-planning with the cooperation and assistance of appropriate state or regional groups. Local health departments and health institutions working with professional societies and community health action-planning groups should assure the development of capabilities for obtaining data necessary for realistic and relevant goal-setting and action-evaluation. Resources for continuing data collection and analysis should be identified, related, utilized, and strengthened as necessary. Personnel with training and competence in data analysis and interpretation should be brought into the action-planning efforts at the very outset. [Page 173]

N-9. Community action-planning groups should seek to increase action research, demonstration, and development of new approaches, especially in health education, data collection and utilization, methods of implementation of action-plans, and organization of community health services. [Page 176]

N-10. The resources of state universities and private institutions of higher learning should be made available to communities to facilitate community health action-planning. [Page 182]

APPENDIX I

History

I. A BRIEF HISTORY OF THE NATIONAL COMMISSION ON COMMUNITY HEALTH SERVICES

Backdrop

The Social Security Act, adopted in the mid-thirties, made available federal grants-in-aid to assist states and communities in the development and financial support of health services. During the next decade, the Congress appropriated health funds to implement this health legislation in various ways. There were no national guidelines for the development of health services until Dr. Haven Emerson and his colleagues published *Health Units for the Nation* in 1945.

The Emerson Report was published by the Commonwealth Fund. Dr. Emerson was chairman of a subcommittee on local health units of the Committee on Administrative Practice of the American Public Health Association (APHA). The report proposed that no population unit or area of the United States remain without a full-time, medically directed health services program responsive to the needs and wishes of the people of the area. It named the following six health services as basic for a local health department: Vital Statistics; Control of Communicable Diseases; Environmental Sanitation; Public Health Laboratory Services; Hygiene of Maternity, Infancy, and Childhood; and Health Education. It estimated that for approximately $1.00 per capita per year it would be possible for a community of 50,000 persons to employ the number and quality of individuals necessary to provide these six basic services.

The Emerson Report was a landmark in the development of public health programs in the United States, but its span of usefulness was short. In the years immediately following 1945, dramatic increase and shifts in population, changes in health needs, planning techniques, and health and medical knowledge radically changed the conditions the Emerson Report had been designed to deal with.

By the mid-fifties, it had become apparent that the very thing that had made the Emerson Report so important at the time of its publication — its firm structural dogma — had actually become a hindrance in meeting the changing health needs of the fluid and mobile community populations of the United States. The force of these changing needs in such a brief period produced chaotic conditions in community health service organization, chiefly in the lack of pattern — particularly in planning — for interagency relations, the lack of effective organization, and the "overlap and gap" in services which stem from these lacks.

The Sponsors. The two major organizations concerned with implementing the report of the Haven Emerson Committee were the APHA and the National Health Council (NHC). The latter staffed the National Advisory Committee on Local Health Departments (NACLHD), and the former worked through its Committee on Public Health Administration and the Subcommittee on Community Public Health Organization. Both had been exploring various possibilities of relating the new and emerging concepts of manpower and health sciences to improved community health services. In April 1958, at an Executive Committee meeting of the NACLHD it was agreed that the Committee's goals should be to stimulate tax-supported local health services and to "needle" the voluntary agencies represented on the Committee to help develop community health services.

Prospectus. The stimulation and the "needling" were effective. By May 1960, a prospectus for a national study of community health services had been developed. It was to be a three-phase study: fact-finding; goal-setting and recommendations; and promotion of local, state, and national action.

Phase One included technical and community fact-finding. The prospectus was not specific as to method, but the fact-finding was to involve all segments of the community. The technical fact-finding was to be the development of basic working papers by selected professional and technical personnel. The community fact-finding would be done at state, regional, and local levels as "a series of probes which would be designed to be helpful in defining needs and providing insights."

Phase Two would be a working conference. This would consist essentially of a national get-together which would examine the product of Phase One activities and seek to establish goals. One product of the conference was to be a final document — a new

"Emerson" Report — together with perhaps several volumes from the various technical and community fact-finding activities.

Phase Three would be marked by the emergence of national, state, and local legislative goals proposals. It would be a period of implementing the fact-finding efforts.

Steering Committee. Late in March 1960, the Executive Committee of the NACLHD named Ernest L. Stebbins, M.D., Chairman of a Steering Committee to develop the proposed project. This Committee met two weeks later to discuss other individuals who might be involved and ways of financing the project.

In March 1961, a contract was negotiated by the APHA with the Public Health Service to provide funds and certain office equipment to staff the development of the proposal for the National Commission on Community Health Services. In May, the Steering Committee, expanded and reconstructed, met to consider the specifics of a proposal, and, in September, the proposal was completed.

The proposal was sent to a group of carefully selected foundations. An application was also made to the Public Health Service. Between December 14, 1961, and March 29, 1962, $920,000 was raised from three sources: The W. K. Kellogg Foundation (a grant of $500,000 over a four-year period); the Public Health Service (a grant of $400,000 over a four-year period); and the McGregor Fund (a grant of $20,000 over a two-year period). Early in May, Marion B. Folsom was named Chairman of the Commission, and later in the same month Dean W. Roberts, M.D., was named Executive Director. During the summer, the staff set up an office in Bethesda, Maryland, and prepared for the first meeting of the Commission.

Organization: Three Projects

The Commission was incorporated under the laws of the state of Maryland on August 28, 1962, and held its first meeting on September 10 and 11. There were 23 Commissioners. At that meeting the Articles of Incorporation and bylaws were ratified, an Executive Committee was elected, a bank account was authorized, a budget was approved, and the officers and Executive Director were authorized to proceed with the work of the Commission.

The Commission's production units were organized as three major projects: National Task Forces, Community Action-Studies, and the National Conference on Community Health Services. This third project later became the Communications Project with the National Conference as one of its functions.

The task forces considered national resources, needs, and trends in terms of community health service potential. The action-studies were conducted in and by communities; their focus was on community problems, utilizing self-study techniques. The National Conference was to provide opportunity for review, discussion, and interpretation of the reports of the other two projects prior to their final publication.

The organizational staff and the production units moved ahead rapidly. By July 1963, four of the task forces authorized by the Commission were fully organized — on Comprehensive Personal Health Services, Environmental Health, Health Care Facilities, and Organization of Community Health Services. Six community action-studies were under way; seven additional communities were submitting applications; and several other communities had indicated interest.

By the end of June 1964, there were 32 Commissioners, and all projects were fully staffed and functioning within the developing plan. A total of 22 communities had been selected, exceeding by 2 the original number planned. The final two task forces, Health Manpower and Financing of Community Health Services and Facilities, had been formed. Conference plans had been formulated, and definite steps were being taken toward the development of a four-forum conference, to be held in September 1965.

The National Task Forces Project

In general, all task forces had the same assignment — to determine how, in the decade ahead, to bring community health services abreast of rapidly changing knowledge and technology for health.

Composition. The task force members were so chosen as to assure the provision of a balance of knowledge and experience in the full range of voluntary and official programs and related interests in the field of community health services, including technical skills and points of view. In the proposal, each task force was to consist of three to five experts in a specific subject area. However, before the first full year of the study was over, the Commission had decided that this was too small a group to provide the range of competence and experience necessary for consideration of such broad subjects as had been assigned to the task forces. Each task force, therefore, consisted of 10 to 15 members. A member of the Commission served with each to facilitate liaison. Consultants were called upon as needed. The chairman of each task force served also as a member of the Advisory Committee to the Project, responsible for over-all coordination among task forces.

Procedures. The work of the task forces was carried out through a series of "work retreat" sessions. These were preceded by an organizational meeting which considered carefully the charge that the task force was given and sought to identify methods of procedure, information, and source materials which would be required, and additional kinds of skills needed. Finally, the meeting set up a timetable. The number of meetings of a task force varied according to the charge, its scope, and the will of the members. For each task force the average number was about eight meetings of approximately three days each. The purpose of the meetings was to develop content and a method of organizing it in relation to the task force charge.

Method of Approach. The essence of the task force operation was to apply knowledge, judgment, experience, and analytical and creative thinking to the assigned subject area, drawing upon presently available information. Primary attention was focused on the organization and administrative aspects of the subject areas rather than on technological features of service programs. Each task force established its own approach to the problem under consideration.

Staff. The central staff consisted of the Director of the Project, the Assistant Director, and an Associate. In addition, each task force had a part-time technical staff to work with the Director of the Project and the Chairman of the Task Force in developing subject-related materials and, eventually, in drafting the reports.

Reports. It was planned that each task force would complete its report no later than June 1965. Prior to this time, drafts of reports would be distributed for review, criticism, and suggestions to the Commission members, the sponsoring agencies, other task forces, technical groups, and selected individuals. The Commission had agreed not to alter the task force reports. This autonomy attracted individuals of the caliber sought by the Commission for its task forces.

The Community Action-Studies Project

Changes in procedure and purpose occurred in both Community Action-Studies and Task Forces Projects. The action-study concept changed from a flat, two-dimensional, fact-finding effort to an exploration of the "dynamics of community health behavior." The project named this exploration "Process Analysis" — a study of the ways in which communities arrived at decisions and took action based on them. Combining self-study with process analysis pointed toward a program of community action-studies which would identify and analyze the principles and methods which facilitate effective community action for the improvement of health services. These studies would test the effectiveness of community self-study. They would also develop ways of enabling community leaders to identify and collect information about their health services and needs, determine priority health goals and establish a plan of action, identify their basic health issues, and stimulate their communities to take effective action to improve health services. The Advisory Committee consisted of 16 members.

Of the 22 communities selected for self-studies, 12 were located east of the Mississippi River, 10 west. Four of the communities had populations in excess of 500,000; 11 between 100,000 and 500,000; and 7 under 100,000. Each of the nine census regions in the United States was represented. There were self-studies in Arkansas, California, Colorado, Idaho, Illinois, Maryland, Massachusetts, Minnesota, Nevada, New Jersey, North Carolina, Ohio, Oklahoma, Oregon, Pennsylvania, South Carolina, Tennessee, Texas, Utah, and Vermont.

The Community Action-Studies Project staff developed a *Planning Guide for the Assessment and Improvement of Community Health Services*. By the end of the second year, the *Planning Guide* was in its third draft and was being used in most of the self-study communities. Consultation to the communities was provided principally through consultants appointed to the communities, who functioned as the Commission's official liaison to them. A combined meeting of all self-study chairmen and coordinators, held May 6, 7, and 8, 1964 in Chattanooga, Tennessee, gave them their first opportunity to discuss together issues and problems facing communities.

Analysis of Previous Studies. This analysis was developed to meet two limitations in the community self-studies activity: the selection of the self-study method from among the other study methods; and the Commission's lack of time (not more than three years) to study the action resulting from the self-studies. Analysis of previous health studies was viewed as a way of broadening this study base and lengthening the time of analysis. A pilot study, made in February 1963, supported the possibility of such an activity and a study proposal was later developed.

Special-Case Studies. Six communities that had experienced unusual success were studied to supplement the project's knowledge of what had been done before: San Mateo County, California; Cincinnati, Ohio; Rochester, New York; Lincoln, Nebraska; Denver, Colorado; and the state of Maryland.

Community Readiness Study. This study was developed to determine why many communities appear to be unready to undertake organized action to solve health problems and to find out what efforts would be necessary to reach and motivate community leaders in general to provide the effective health leadership necessary. A pilot study, undertaken in November 1963, clarified concepts used in the study.

The Communications Project

By the end of 1964, the Communications Project had been able to define its activity as a running dialogue with selected groups or with individuals to help accomplish the Commission's purposes and arrive at its goals. The project had developed a system to direct and coordinate the Commission's contribution to the dialogue.

The communications functions were planned to make available to Commission leadership, Sponsors, Commissioners, and Advisory Committees the information and knowledge they required to direct the Commission's work, to provide a continuous flow of information among production units to coordinate their efforts, to maintain an exchange of information among communities conducting studies with Commission assistance and among other communities conducting similar studies without Commission assistance, and to inform and receive information from the Commission's various publics.

The Communications Project set up meetings, distributed reports of program progress, arranged for Commissioners and other Commission leadership to make speeches and participate with other groups in discussions of the Commission's work, and planned for a National Conference for creative review and discussion of the Commission's reports. The Commission also had begun to use a wide variety of communications channels, including libraries, conferences, seminars, speakers bureaus, the Community Health *Newsletter*, technological journals, press, radio, and TV. An Advisory Committee to the Project had been appointed, as had a National Conference Planning Committee, both staffed by the Communications Project.

The National Conference. By the end of 1964, the Conference Planning Committee had developed plans for a four-forum conference in September 1965, to meet in San Francisco, Chicago, Atlanta, and Philadelphia in sequent weeks. Its purpose had been described as getting reactions to the Commission's recommendations and findings in terms of feasibility, acceptability, usefulness, and vision. Participants were to be invited. The Planning Committee anticipated an attendance of 300 people at each of the Conferences. The National Conference was to be the National Health Council Forum for 1965. There was to be a fifth forum in the early spring of 1966, which would be national and which would concern itself primarily with the Commission Report.

The Community Action-Studies Project assembled its study chairmen and coordinators in New York for a meeting in mid-December. This was an expansion of the May 1964 meeting in Chattanooga, in that Commission staff, Commissioners, and the Advisory Committee met with representatives of all of the community studies. It provided all participants with an opportunity to express concern, question concepts and procedures, and react to the Commission's plans.

After the first of January 1965, the Commission concerned itself primarily with the Reports and the Conference, which had been set for September 1965.

Reports

The six task forces prepared provisional drafts of their reports for use at the regional forums by July 1965. The recommendations covered wide areas of content: financing, staffing, and housing for both environmental and personal health services, and the kinds of resources available and necessary and ways to organize them to deliver the necessary health services.

The Community Action-Studies Project had received interim reports from its four basic research activities. One of the 22 communities had begun its self-study organization but decided it could not continue. Of the 21 communities participating, 3 had completed their studies and had published reports, 7 had completed their studies and had reports in process, and the remaining 11 were at various stages of their study process. The fourth and final revision of the *Planning Guide* was under way. The Commonwealth Fund had agreed to subsidize publication of the Commission's reports.

The Conference

The Conference plan had been approved and four regional forum committees had been developed to assist in selecting the participants for the forums. As plans for the forums were developed, two instruments were produced to facilitate its purposes: a reaction sheet and the Conference Workbook. From January until September 1965, almost the entire work of the Commission was devoted to the development of these two instruments.

Reaction Sheet. The reaction sheet was devised to test the Commission's recommendations by regions and by individuals. The following tests were applied to each recommendation: Can it be done? Would it be useful if it were done? Would it be acceptable? Does it look to the future? Each participant evaluated the recommendations in terms of the four tests, the reaction sheets were machine tabulated, and their messages analyzed.

Workbook. The workbook was an organization of the recommendations and findings of the two study projects for discussion purposes. It contained the recommendations and summary statements with a minimum of connective tissue. Every conferee had one in advance of the forum he attended.

Committee on the Commission Report. In May, a committee of four Commissioners had been appointed to plan and supervise the preparation of the Commission Report. In mid-August, the committee involved the entire Commission in developing a set of imperatives taken from the task force recommendations and community action-studies. In three days of exciting work, a set of 49 imperatives — not recommendations, but activities which would be essential to the delivery of community health services — were dredged from the project reports.

The Final Year

Task Forces. The task forces met in New York City in November to consider the reaction of the regional forums. One of the results of this meeting was that the number of recommendations was reduced by eliminating what were regarded as the less significant ones and by combining others. Task Force reports were then revised in line with instructions from the task forces at the November meeting and with consultation from task force chairmen. All of them were scheduled for submitting to the publisher by June 1966.

Community Studies. The CASP Advisory Committee met after the Conference also and outlined its own report. Data on all but one of the research projects were expected by February 1966. By April, a draft of the CASP Report was sent to Committee members, and final reports on all phases of CASP's activities were scheduled for completion by fall.

The Commission Report. The Commission Report, however, which had been developed only to the point of a set of imperatives in August, now began to demand special concern. At meetings of the Committee on the Report and the full Commission, Commissioners sought to check the imperatives against Conference reactions, establish a priority among the imperatives, determine any serious omissions, and develop basic positions and recommendations. By December 29, 1965, a first draft of the Report had been completed, and the Commission approved the final draft in March 1966.

The Report, called *Health Is a Community Affair*, was released to the public on April 22, 1966. Marion B. Folsom, as Chairman of the Commission, presented it to President Lyndon B. Johnson at a ceremony in the Cabinet Room of the White House. In his presentation, Mr. Folsom stated his wish that this affair "may prosper in communities all over the land." He said that the Commission looked forward to the time when "every resident of the nation, whether he lives in New York City, the West Virginia hills, the bayous of Louisiana or the plains, mountain or coastal areas of the country, should be able to learn about and attain those health services needful to himself, his family and his neighbors."

President Johnson accepted the report for all the people of the United States. He called the recommendations exciting, and said that they confronted the problems "that we must, in time, face up to." Referring to replacement of scarce personnel in hospitals and the resultant higher hospital costs, the President said: "a tax bill won't change that situation much, and a control bill won't change that situation much." He accented the need for trained people rather than legislation: "We are going to have to have more people trained in this [health] field." He said that American manpower is not organized to provide effective service: "Our age, which is an age of miracles, is still an age where too many families must travel too far and pay too much to receive treatment, where health services are not organized to get the full benefit of our health manpower."

The Commission Report formed the basis for the 1966 National Health Forum of the National Health Council, held in New York City on May 9–11. The Forum theme was: Action for Comprehensive Health Services — the Implication of Recommendations of the National Commission on Community Health Services. More than 600 community leaders, many of whom had played a part in developing the Report, attended this Forum. Their use of the Report and their endorsement of its recommendations assured the Commission that its time and effort had been well invested.

Personnel

STEERING COMMITTEE ON COMMUNITY HEALTH SERVICES*

Ernest L. Stebbins, M.D., M.P.H., Chairman

Margaret G. Arnstein, R.N., M.P.H.
George W. Cooley
Howard W. Ennes, M.P.H.
Vlado A. Getting, M.D., Dr.P.H.
Sam A. Kimble

J. W. R. Norton, M.D., M.P.H.
James E. Perkins, M.D., Dr.P.H.
James K. Shafer, M.D., M.P.H.
Charles L. Wilbar, Jr., M.D.
Franklin D. Yoder, M.D., M.P.H.

Ex-officio Committee Members

Thomas R. Hood, M.D., M.P.H.
George James, M.D., M.P.H.
Berwyn F. Mattison, M.D., M.P.H.

Peter G. Meek
Levitte Mendel, M.P.H., M.S.P.H.
John D. Porterfield, M.D., M.P.H.

NATIONAL COMMISSION ON COMMUNITY HEALTH SERVICES

Officers

Marion B. Folsom, M.B.A., LL.D., Chairman
Director, Eastman Kodak Company
James E. Perkins, M.D., Dr.P.H., Vice-Chairman
Managing Director, National Tuberculosis Association
Joseph L. Beesley, C.L.U., Treasurer
Senior Vice-President and Assistant to Chairman,
Equitable Life Assurance Society of the United States
Dean W. Roberts, M.D., M.P.H., Secretary
Executive Director, National Commission on
Community Health Services

* This group guided the development of the proposal for the National Commission on Community Health Services.

Commissioners

C. H. Hardin Branch, M.D., Chairman, Department of Psychiatry, University of Utah College of Medicine

Leroy E. Burney, M.D., M.P.H., Vice-President for Health Sciences, Temple University

LeRoy Collins, LL.B., Under Secretary of Commerce

Edwin L. Crosby, M.D., Dr.P.H., Executive Vice-President and Director, American Hospital Association

Nelson H. Cruikshank, B.D., Director, Department of Social Security, AFL-CIO

Albert W. Dent, LL.D., President, Dillard University

Fairleigh S. Dickinson, Jr., President, Becton, Dickinson and Company

Milton Stover Eisenhower, LL.D., D.Sc., President, The Johns Hopkins University

Stanford F. Farnsworth, M.D., M.P.H., Director, Maricopa County Health Department

James A. Hamilton, M.C.S., Director of Hospital Administration, University of Minnesota

Harry G. Hanson, M.S., Assistant Surgeon General, Public Health Service, United States Department of Health, Education, and Welfare

Herman E. Hilleboe, M.D., M.P.H., DeLamar Professor of Public Health Practice, Columbia University School of Public Health and Administrative Medicine

Harold A. James, Ph.B., LL.B., Attorney-at-Law, Doyle, Lewis and Warner

Boisfeuillet Jones, B.Ph., LL.B., President, Emily and Ernest Woodruff Foundation

John W. Knutson, D.D.S., Dr.P.H., Professor of Preventive Dentistry and Public Health, University of California, Los Angeles

Sanford P. Lehman, M.D., M.P.H., Director of Health, Seattle-King County Health Department

Berwyn F. Mattison, M.D., M.P.H. (ex officio), Executive Director, The American Public Health Association

William F. McGlone, LL.B., Attorney-at-Law, Denver, Colorado

Walter J. McNerney, M.H.A., President, Blue Cross Association

Joseph H. McNinch, M.D., Chief Medical Director, Department of Medicine and Surgery, Veterans Administration

Peter G. Meek (ex officio), Executive Director, National Health Council

Marion W. Sheahan, R.N., Deputy General Director, National League for Nursing, Inc.

Charles D. Shields, M.D., M.P.H., Chairman, Department of Physical Medicine and Rehabilitation, University of Vermont College of Medicine

Charles E. Smith, M.D., D.P.H., Dean, School of Public Health, University of California, Berkeley

Virginia Dodd Smith, Deputy President of Associated Country Women of the World (1962)

William C. Treuhaft, L.H.D., President, Tremco Manufacturing Company

John H. Venable, M.D., M.P.H., Director, Georgia Department of Public Health

Raymond L. White, M.D., Consultant on Socioeconomic Activities to the Executive Vice-President, American Medical Association

Jane E. Wrieden, M.S.W., National Consultant, Women's and Children's Services, the Salvation Army National Headquarters

PROJECT ADVISORY COMMITTEES

National Task Forces Project

Ernest L. Stebbins, M.D., M.P.H., Chairman

Gaylord W. Anderson, M.D., Dr.P.H.	George James, M.D., M.P.H.
	Leonard W. Mayo, S.Sc.D.
Ray E. Brown, M.B.A., H.H.D.	Isidor S. Ravdin, M.D., L.H.D.,
Richard W. Case, LL.B.	LL.D.
Lenor S. Goerke, M.D., M.S.P.H.	

Community Action-Studies Project

Hugh R. Leavell, M.D., Chairman until May 1963
George James, M.D., M.P.H., Chairman

Jesse B. Aronson, M.D., M.P.H.	Merrill F. Krughoff, M.A.
Wallace H. Best, Ph.D.	Sewall Milliken, M.P.H.
Clarissa E. Boyd, M.P.H.	Irwin M. Rosenstock, Ph.D.
George Bugbee, A.B.	Robert A. Sigmond, M.A.
Howard Ennes, M.P.H.	Raymond L. White, M.D.
Vlado A. Getting, M.D., Dr.P.H.	Theodore D. Woolsey
Ira V. Hiscock, Sc.D., M.P.H.	Wesley O. Young, D.M.D., M.P.H.
Robert C. Hoover, Ph.D.	

Communications Project

> LeRoy Collins, LL.B., Chairman until May 1964
> A. H. Thiemann, Chairman

Richard Bernstein   J. Stewart Hunter
John M. Couric   Miss Dallas Johnson
Edward L. Greif   Robert Yoho, H.S.D.
James E. Hague

NATIONAL TASK FORCES

Task Force on Environmental Health

> Gaylord W. Anderson, M.D., Dr.P.H., Chairman

Clark D. Ahlberg, Ph.D.   Harold M. Erickson, M.D.,
Philip S. Broughton   M.P.H.
Robert M. Brown, P.E.   Harry G. Hanson, M.S.
Charles E. Carl, M.S.   P. Walton Purdom, M.G.A., Ph.D.
C. Howe Eller, M.D., Dr.P.H.   Meredith H. Thompson, Dr.Eng.

Task Force on Comprehensive Personal Health Services

> Isidor S. Ravdin, M.D., L.H.D., LL.D., Chairman

Daniel Blain, M.D.   Norvin C. Kiefer, M.D., M.P.H.
Lester Breslow, M.D., M.P.H.   Granville W. Larimore, M.D.,
Robin C. Buerki, M.D.   M.P.H.
Leroy E. Burney, M.D., M.P.H.   Carl L. Sebelius, D.D.S., M.P.H.
John L. Caughey, Jr., M.D.   Marion W. Sheahan, R.N.
Melvin A. Glasser, LL.D.   William H. Stewart, M.D.
Charles L. Hudson, M.D.   Myron E. Wegman, M.D.

Task Force on Health Manpower

> Lenor S. Goerke, M.D., M.S.P.H., Chairman

Harold D. Chope, M.D., Dr.P.H.   Glen R. Leymaster, M.D., M.P.H.
Stanford F. Farnsworth, M.D.,   Marion I. Murphy, Ph.D., M.P.H.
  M.P.H.   Paul J. Sanazaro, M.D.
John W. Knutson, D.D.S., Dr.P.H.   Frank M. Stead, M.S.
Robert H. Kroepsch, Ed.D.   George Wheatley, M.D., M.P.H.

Task Force on Health Care Facilities

Ray E. Brown, M.B.A., H.H.D., Chairman

John B. Atwater, M.D., Dr.P.H.
William E. Beaumont, Jr.
Jack C. Haldeman, M.D., M.P.H.
Daniel Lieberman, M.D.
David Littauer, M.D.
Elisabeth C. Phillips, R.N.

Delbert L. Pugh
John M. Rumsey, M.D.
Carl K. Schmidt, Jr., Ph.B.
William A. Spencer, M.D.
Nathan J. Stark, LL.D.
John H. Venable, M.D., M.P.H.

Task Force on Financing Community Health Services and Facilities

Richard W. Case, LL.B., Chairman

Clark D. Ahlberg, Ph.D.
Lisbeth Bamberger
Richard C. Brockway
C. Manton Eddy
Milton S. Eisenhower, LL.D.,
    D.Sc.
Lyman S. Ford

James A. Maxwell, Ph.D.
Russell A. Nelson, M.D.
T. Eric Reynolds, M.A., M.D.
Wilson T. Sowder, M.D., M.P.H.
Alexander L. Stott
Russell E. Teague, M.D., M.P.H.
James A. Walsh, M.D.

Task Force on Organization of Community Health Services

Leonard W. Mayo, S.Sc.D., Chairman

Philip D. Bonnet, M.D.
James Brindle
Nathaniel H. Cooper, M.D.,
    M.P.H.
Herman E. Hilleboe, M.D.,
    M.P.H.

Roscoe P. Kandle, M.D., M.P.H.
William J. Peeples, M.D., M.P.H.
Alfred M. Popma, M.D.
John H. Romani
Walter Wenkert, M.P.H.
Alonzo S. Yerby, M.D., M.P.H.

COMMUNITY SELF-STUDY LEADERS

Arkansas: Ouachita County–Camden
  Perry Dalton, M.D., Chairman
  Coy Dildy, Coordinator
  Mrs. Marie Broach, P.H.N., Assistant Coordinator
California: San Mateo County
  Elwood Ennis, Chairman
  Hope Spencer, M.P.H., Coordinator

Idaho: Idaho Falls
  Ivan Miller, Chairman (until 1965)
  Seth L. Jenkins, Chairman
  Robert Steiling, Coordinator
Illinois: Sangamon County–Springfield
  Emmett F. Pearson, M.D., Chairman (until 1965)
  William De Hollander, M.D., Chairman
  Mrs. Virginia Ostermeier, Coordinator
Maryland: Prince George's County
  Mrs. William H. Wood, Chairman
  Miss Betty Gredig, M.P.H., Coordinator
Massachusetts: Springfield
  Herbert P. Almgren, Chairman
  Robert J. Van Wart, M.S.W., Coordinator
  Hamp Coley, M.P.H., Assistant Coordinator
Minnesota: St. Louis County–Duluth
  Fred Lewis, Chairman
  John Dilley, M.P.H., Coordinator
Nevada: Reno–Washoe County
  Richard Brown, M.D., Chairman
  Robert Seach, Coordinator
New Jersey: Cape May County
  Robert J. Fitzpatrick, Chairman
  Sybil Buffman, Coordinator (until 1964)
  Mildred Patterson, M.S.P.H., Coordinator
New Jersey: Newark
  Harry W. Jones, Chairman
  Leo Kaye, M.A., Coordinator (until 1965)
  Lt. Col. George B. Warren, Jr., Coordinator
North Carolina: Halifax County
  Paul Johnston, Chairman
  Ralph Kilby, M.D., M.P.H., Coordinator (until 1964)
  Robert Young, M.D., M.P.H., Coordinator
  Mrs. Lois Batton, Assistant Coordinator
Ohio: Toledo–Lucas County
  Robert Knight, Chairman
  Mary V. Hayes, M.P.H., Coordinator (until 1965)
  James Pullella, M.P.H., Coordinator
Oklahoma: Enid–Garfield County
  Ralph Goley, Co-chairman
  John McMillan, Co-chairman
  James Price, Coordinator

Oregon: Lane County–Eugene
  Donald Brinton, M.D., Chairman (until 1965)
  Harold Johnson, Jr., Chairman
  Miriam L. Tuck, Ed.D., Coordinator
  Mrs. Johnnye Schick, R.N., Assistant Coordinator
Pennsylvania: Bucks County
  John B. Leedom, Chairman
  Walter Baily, M.S.W., Coordinator
South Carolina: Charleston
  Edward Kronsberg, Chairman
  Mrs. Irene Burnett, Coordinator (until 1965)
  Charles Fruit, Coordinator
Tennessee: Chattanooga
  William G. Brown, Chairman
  George Rice, M.S.W., Coordinator
  Wood C. McCue, M.P.H., Assistant Coordinator
Tennessee: Knox Area
  Wilbur Roos, Chairman (until 1964)
  J. T. Mengel, Chairman
  T. E. Wintersteen, M.S.W., Coordinator
Texas: San Antonio
  A. P. Thaddeus, M.D., Chairman
  Olin W. LeBaron, M.S.W., Coordinator
Utah: Salt Lake City
  Joseph Rosenblatt, Chairman (until 1965)
  H. C. Shoemaker, Chairman
  Eva Hancock, Coordinator (until 1965)
  William M. Stewart, Coordinator
  Robert K. Ward, Associate Coordinator
Vermont: Burlington
  William L. Wright, Chairman, Steering Committee
  Mrs. Ethan A. Sims, Chairman, Advisory Committee
  Alfred Haynes, M.D., M.P.H., Coordinator (until 1964)
  Mrs. E. Grafton Carlisle, Coordinator

NATIONAL CONFERENCE ON COMMUNITY
HEALTH SERVICES, 1965

Conference Planning Committee

Charles E. Smith, M.D., D.P.H., Chairman, 1963–64
William C. Treuhaft, L.H.D., Chairman, 1964–65

Edwin L. Crosby, M.D., Dr.P.H.   Albert W. Dent, LL.D.
Berwyn F. Mattison, M.D.,   Peter G. Meek
M.P.H.   Marion W. Sheahan, R.N.

Forum Leaders

San Francisco

Roy Sorenson and Malcolm H. Merrill, M.D., Regional Committee
Chairmen
John W. Knutson, D.D.S., Dr.P.H., Forum Chairman
Arthur S. Flemming, LL.D., L.H.D., Keynote Speaker

Chicago

Harold Hillenbrand, D.D.S., Regional Committee Chairman
Edwin L. Crosby, M.D., Dr.P.H., Forum Chairman
Charles H. Percy, LL.D., L.H.D., Keynote Speaker

Atlanta

Edgar J. Forio, LL.B., Regional Committee Chairman
John W. Venable, M.D., M.P.H., Forum Chairman
Edgar J. Forio, LL.B., Keynote Speaker

Philadelphia

Isidor S. Ravdin, M.D., Regional Committee Chairman
Leroy E. Burney, M.D., M.P.H., Forum Chairman
John E. Fogarty, Keynote Speaker

COMMISSION STAFF

Central Staff

Dean W. Roberts, M.D., M.P.H., Executive Director
Aaron L. Andrews, M.P.H., Assistant Executive Director for Administration
Mrs. Cozette H. Barker, M.P.H., Assistant Director, National Task
Forces Project
Walter M. Beattie, Jr., M.A., Director, National Task Forces Project
Walter R. Cuskey, M.S.W., Staff Associate (July 1963–August 1965)
Mrs. Lue Faris, Assistant to the Director, Community Action-Studies
Project (August 1962–December 1964)
Clyde C. Hall, Editor
Miss Hazel Holly, Writer
Lee Holder, M.P.H., Director, Community Action-Studies Project

Paul R. Mico, M.A., M.P.H., Director, Community Action-Studies Project (September 1962–December 1964)

Robert Parrish, M.A., Director of Publications (February 1963–March 1964)

Perry F. Prather, M.D., Special Consultant to the Executive Director

T. Lefoy Richman, M.A., Assistant Executive Director for Communications and Director, Communications Project

Mrs. Clara Schiffer, M.A., Statistical Analyst (March 1963–January 1964)

Richard H. Schlesinger, M.P.H., M.S.W., Associate Director, National Task Forces Project

Mrs. Wanda Van Goor, M.A., Director of Publications

Staff Associates

Thomas R. Hood, M.D., M.P.H., American Public Health Association

Levitte Mendel, M.P.H., M.S.P.H., National Health Council

Technical Staff, Consultants, and Sponsor Representatives to the National Task Forces Project

W. H. Aufranc, M.D., M.P.H.

Richard G. Bond, M.S., M.P.H.

Wesley E. Gilbertson, B.S.E.E., M.S.P.H.

Arthur J. Grimes, M.P.H.

Thomas E. Hanrahan, M.S.

William L. Kissick, M.D., Dr.P.H.

Herbert E. Klarman, Ph.D.

George J. Kupchik, Dr.Eng.

Darrel J. Mase, Ph.D.

Basil J. F. Mott, M.P.A.

Robert J. Mowitz, Ph.D.

Mrs. Maryland Pennell, M.S.

Leo G. Reeder, Ph.D.

Mrs. Ruth Roemer, LL.B.

Richard Sasuly, M.A.

Howard N. Schulz, B.S.

Hiram Sibley, M.S., M.A.

William A. Spencer, M.D.

Matthew Tayback, Sc.D.

William C. Thomas, Ph.D.

Technical Staff, Consultants, and Sponsor Representatives to the Community Action-Studies Project

Robert E. Agger, Ph.D., LL.B.

Jesse B. Aronson, M.D., M.P.H.

Floyd C. Beelman, M.D.

Heinrik L. Blum, M.D., M.P.H.

George Robert Boynton, Ph.D.

Robert Paul Boynton, Ph.D.

Robert M. Brown

Robert E. Coker, M.D., M.P.H.

Ralph W. Conant, Ph.D.

O. Lynn Deniston, M.P.H.

Richard G. Domey, Ed.D.

Harold M. Erickson, M.D., M.P.H.

Stanford F. Farnsworth, M.D., M.P.H.

J. T. Gentry, M.D., M.P.H.

Vlado A. Getting, M.D., Dr.P.H.
Marshall N. Goldstein, Ph.D.
Donald P. Haefner, Ph.D.
Thomas E. Hanrahan, M.S.
Herman E. Hilleboe, M.D.,
  M.P.H.
Thomas R. Hood, M.D., M.P.H.
Lee Holder, M.P.H.
S. Stephen Kegeles, Ph.D.
George M. Keranen, M.D., M.P.H.
Merrill F. Krughoff, M.A.
Ronald Lippitt, Ph.D.
W. Frederick Mayes, M.D.,
  M.P.H.
Cyrus Mayshark, H.S.D.
William C. McCue, M.P.H.

Gordon McGregor, Ph.D.
Sewall Milliken, M.P.H.
Robert Morris, Ph.D.
Perry F. Prather, M.D.
Edward Press, M.D., M.P.H.
Kim Rodner, Ph.D.
Peter Rossi, Ph.D.
Bradbury Seasholes, Ph.D.
Erwin Scheuch, Ph.D.
Howard Slusher, Ph.D.
Peter G. Snow, Ph.D.
Michael Springer
Bert E. Swanson, Ph.D.
Richard L. Wenzel, M.D., M.P.H.
Robert N. Wilson, Ph.D.

Technical Staff and Consultants to the Conference Planning Committee

Howard Ennes, M.P.H.
Arthur J. Grimes, M.P.H.
Michael E. McMahon

William L. Kissick, M.D., Dr.P.H.
William P. McCahill

Index

(Letters and numbers in bold face indicate that the Commission took a position or made a recommendation on the subject and refer to the number of that position or recommendation and the pages on which it is found.)

ference on Community Health Services, 232; reaction sheet, 233
Constitution of the United States, *re* state power, 128
Congress, 88th, 89th, 194
Consumer: health services, 53, 56; education (E-10, E-11), 68, 69, 207, 208; protection (E-10), 69, 208; costs, 70; Social Security, 75, 76; care, 188
Continuing education: medical (C-2, C-4), 25, 27, 203, 205; health training institutions and (J-18), 27, 215; in health resources and services (I), 27, 211; in health training, 99; for pathologists, 100
Continuity, of care, 54, 134
Contracts, for health services, 136
Controversy, 181, 182
Coordination: in health facilities (K-6), 113, 216; (N-2), 170, 221
Coordinator, role in planning, 87
Costs: of quackery, 67; State of Maryland Commission to Study Hospital Costs, 104; of hospital care (K, K-5), 111, 215–216; pro-rata allocation of, 114; New York Governor's Committee report, 115; in rural areas, 122. *See also* Hospital
Council on Dental Health, American Dental Association, 36
Counseling and referral service (B-3), 29, 200
Criteria: developing, Health, Education, and Welfare, 60; to measure effect of urban living (H-2), 60, 210; for manpower training (J-4), 82, 212; National Health Council, 164
Crowding, effects of (H-1), 59, 210
Cultists, 67
Curriculum: community psychiatry in medical schools, 35; in medical schools, 94; need for community medicine in, 94; for health planners (N-7), 172, 222

Data: collecting and processing (N-8), 54, 55, 112, 135, 143, 173, 222; sources (N-8), 173, 222
Deaths: causes, 5, 91; certification by medical examiner, 91
Delegation: of nonmedical health care (C-1), 22, 203; of health functions (L-5), 141, 218
Dental Health, 35, 36
Dental schools, auxiliary personnel in (J-6), 86, 213

Dentists: in personal health services, 30; number of, 80, 81
Discrimination, racial: as manpower waste (J-11), 94, 213
Drugs, 146

Education: of personal physician, 26–27; in health resources (I), 62, 211; in pollution (E-11), 69, 208; strengthening, 93; continuity of, 179
Education for health, individual responsibility (I), 62, 210; community responsibility (I), 62, 211; in business and industry (I-2), 64, 211; school curriculums (I-1), 64, 211; in public health schools (I-5), 66, 84, 211; research findings (I-3), 66, 211; training personnel (I-4), 66, 211
Emerson, Haven, *Health Units for the Nation*, 225
Emergency services, 118, 119
Enforcement authority, state as (L-3), 140, 218
Environment: meaning, 38, 39; crisis in, 39; control of (E), 39, 78, 89, 205, 206; a totality, 40; public health agency, responsibility for (E-1), 40, 206; research in, 41; hazards, 78, 89
Environmental health services inseparable from personal services, 7; (A-1, D), 38, 130, 197, 205; manpower in, 41; Public Health Service, 41; personnel, qualifications, 89; team approach, 89; task force on, 228. *See also* National Task Forces
Epidemiology, 91
"Expediter," 87

Family: planning (G), 57–58, 209; disorganization, 58; research (G-1), 58, 209; instruction in (G-2), 58, 209
Federal government: in regulation of chemicals (E), 12, 208; financial support of health services, 15, 188 (L-7), 147, 218–219; legislation, 142; grants for public health, 146
Financing health services (B-10), 71, 74, 201; (J-14), 94, 96, 214; state and public, 133, (L-3, L-6), 140, 142, 218; local health units, 141, 142, 218; federal support (L-7), 147, 218, 219; long-range planning (N-4), 170, 221; private funds for, 187–188. *See also* Grants
Financing of Community Health Services and Facilities, 228. *See also* National Task Forces